A patient's guide and explanations of

Breast cancer treatment

Prepared by

Dr. Badria Eid Al-Johani

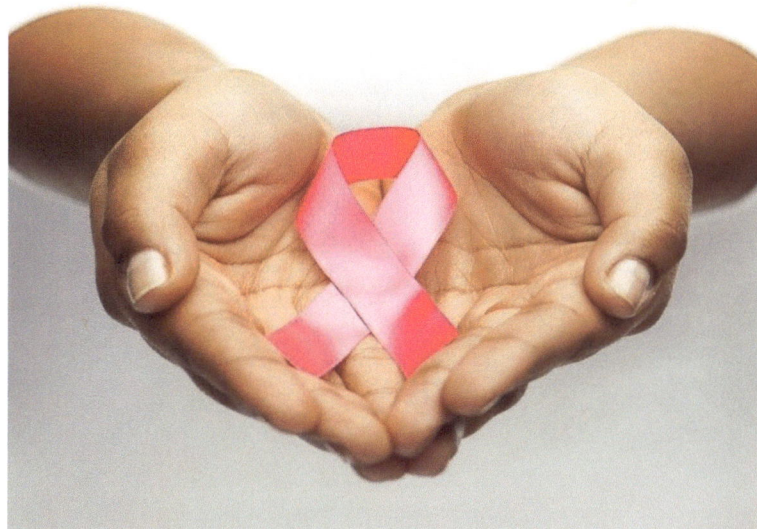

**This guidebook is considered as your reference of your treatment.
Please bring it with you to each clinic visit and use the drawing and note
space in the back to document your treatment plan and questions.**

A patient's guide and explanations of Breast cancer treatment

A patient's guide and explanations of Breast cancer treatment

Dr. Badria Eid Al-Johani

Consultant General Surgery

Consultant Breast and Endocrine Oncology Surgery

A patient's guide and explanations of Breast cancer treatment

A patient's guide and explanations of Breast cancer treatment

Written by

Dr. Badria Eid Al-Johani
Consultant General Surgery
Consultant Breast & Endocrine Surgery

ISBN 978-0-9909322-0-8

Printed on Demand by Createspace.com
Distributed by Amazon and Internationale affiliates

Contact Eid & Otto Internationale
info@eid-otto.com

visit us at
http://www.eid-otto.com

Eid & Otto Internationale
1712 Pioneer Ave, Suite 670
Cheyenne, WY, 82001
USA

1-405-287-8227

A patient's guide and explanations of Breast cancer treatment

A patient's guide and explanations of Breast cancer treatment

TABLE OF CONTENTS

A patient's guide and explanations of Breast cancer treatment

A patient's guide and explanations of Breast cancer treatment

Introduction

Breast cancer is the most common cancer among females all over the world. Many women die annually with advanced breast cancer due to delay in diagnosis and treatment.

It is important to know that breast cancer is a disease that can be cured in the early stages by screening and early doctor consultation.

Breast cancer is possible in men although at a significantly lower rate. The treatments and surgeries are the same as women.

In this guide, we discuss and explain the treatment plan for each patient diagnosed with breast cancer and what she can expect as patient before and after surgery.

A patient's guide and explanations of Breast cancer treatment

ANATOMY OF THE BREAST

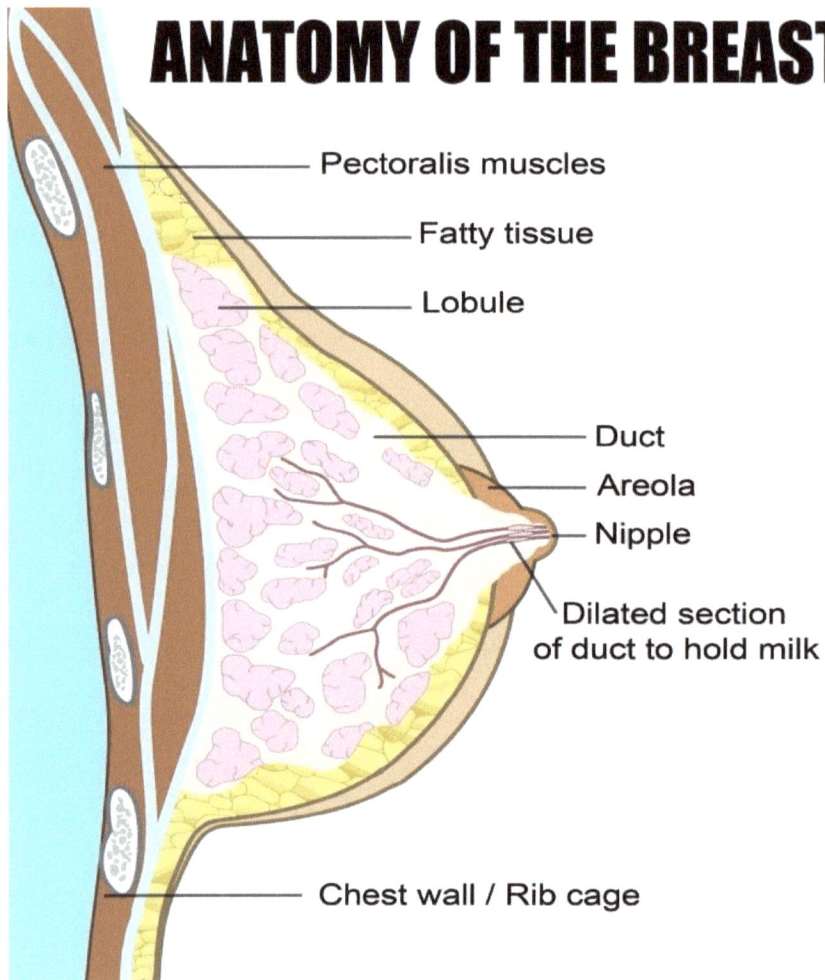

Pectoralis muscles

Fatty tissue

Lobule

Duct

Areola

Nipple

Dilated section
of duct to hold milk

Chest wall / Rib cage

Before beginning to describe the anatomy of the breast, know that every woman's body is unique and different. Every woman's breasts are also unique and different, there is no absolute model of what a breast is, or should be or must be.

Anatomy of the breast

The breast is located on the top of chest wall; both breasts are similar in shape and location, often with very mild differences. The breast generally extends from midline of the chest to the Axilla (Axillary tail also called 'breast tail'). The shape of breast is generally a teardrop form with variation from conical in women with no children to pendulous in women with children.

The size of breast is variable according to fat distribution in the body, the breast increases or decreases in size depending on the amount of fat in the body.

Each breast consisted of 15-20 parts (segments) separated by fibrous tissue. Each segment has glands; each gland has lobules, where the milk is formed, and duct which is tube like, where the milk is drained through to the main duct then to the nipple into separate orifice. It is important to observe if you have a nipple discharge to know which orifice is the discharge is coming from.

The breast contains blood vessels that bring oxygen and nutrients to breast, lymphatic channels and lymph nodes as part of immune system.

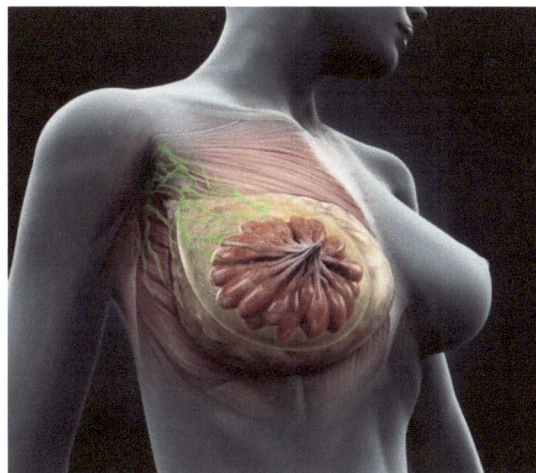

A patient's guide and explanations of Breast cancer treatment

7

Lymphatic drainage of the breast

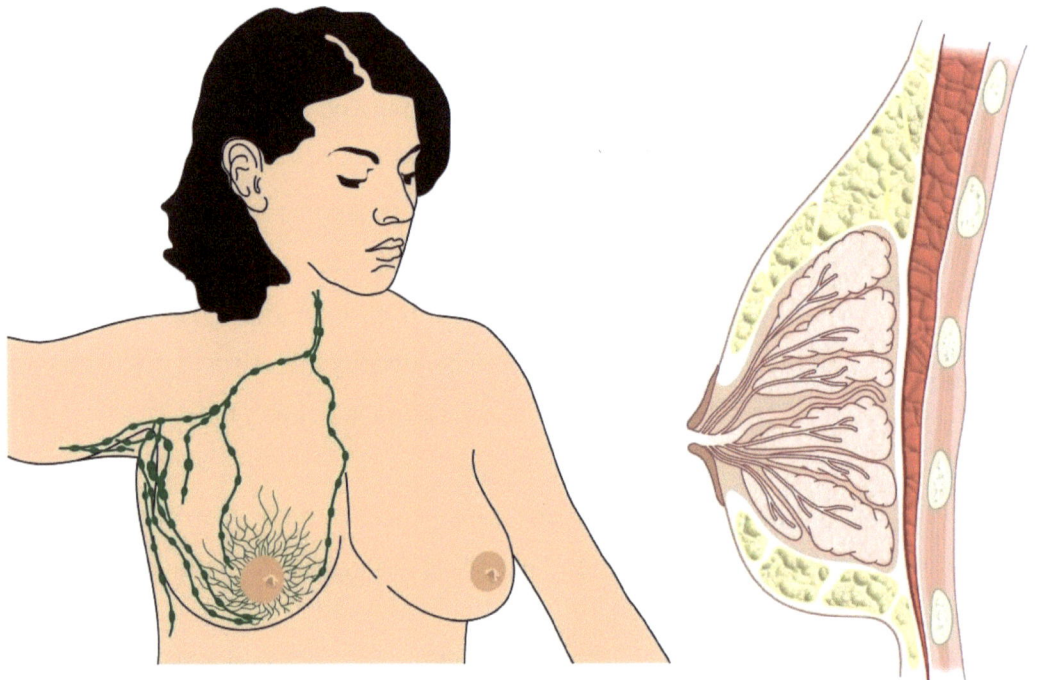

Approximately 75% of lymphatic drainage of breast is going through lymphatic vessels to Axillary lymph nodes which are located in the arm pit, and 25% are going to lymph node in the middle of the breast bone.

The lymph nodes in the arm pit can receive lymphatic drainage from the arm and any disturbance in the lymph nodes under the arm pit it may lead to swelling of the arm called *lymphedema* (lim-fo-ed-ee-mah)

A patient's guide and explanations of Breast cancer treatment

Breast cancer presentations

The term "presentation" means the things that you or your family doctor have noticed, discovered or suspect before or at the time of your initial breast clinic visit.

- **Breast lump**

Most of the patients with breast cancer visit the doctor for the first time when they find a breast lump. Self-breast examination is important for early detection of breast cancer leading to a better outcome.

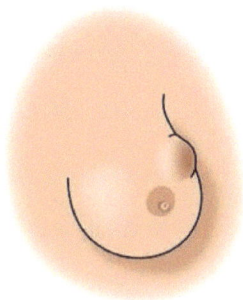

- **Skin changes**

The skin covering the breast can also indicate changes.   These can be in many variations from reddening, dimpling, 'orange skin' like characteristics, to skin ulceration and tumor fungation with foul smelling discharge. ('Orange skin' refers to the porous outer peel of the orange citrus fruit, not the color).

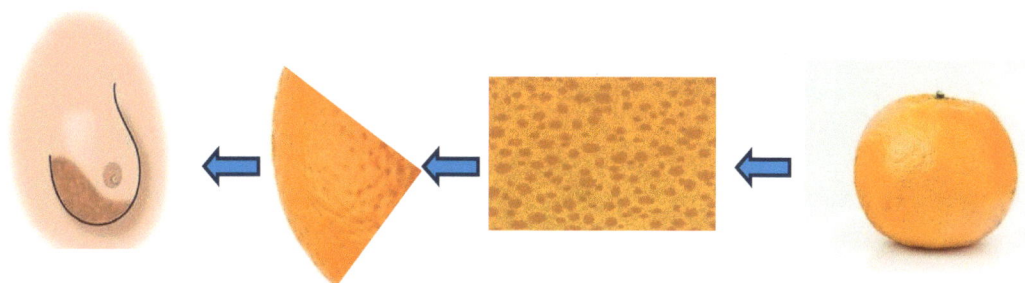

A patient's guide and explanations of Breast cancer treatment

Breast cancer presentations (continue)

- **Nipple-areola changes**

Nipple-areola change is a very significant alarm for malignancy, mainly if the change is newly developed, for example: nipple retraction, nipple deviation, areola excoriation or eczema like changes (Paget's disease)

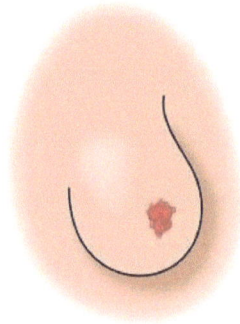

- **Nipple discharge**

One of sign of breast cancer is nipple discharge, <u>but is it important to notice the color of the discharge, content, and which orifice in the nipple</u>. Early cancer needs to be excluded.

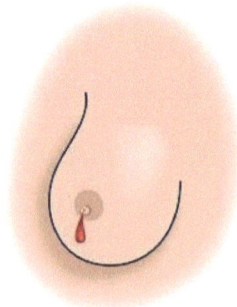

Breast cancer presentations (continue)

- ## Armpit lump

Some patients may develop breast cancer at the armpit or Breast tail (part of breast - under arm pit, or Axillary lymph nodes).Enlargement likely indicates metastases (spreading) of cancer cells to Axillary lymph node.

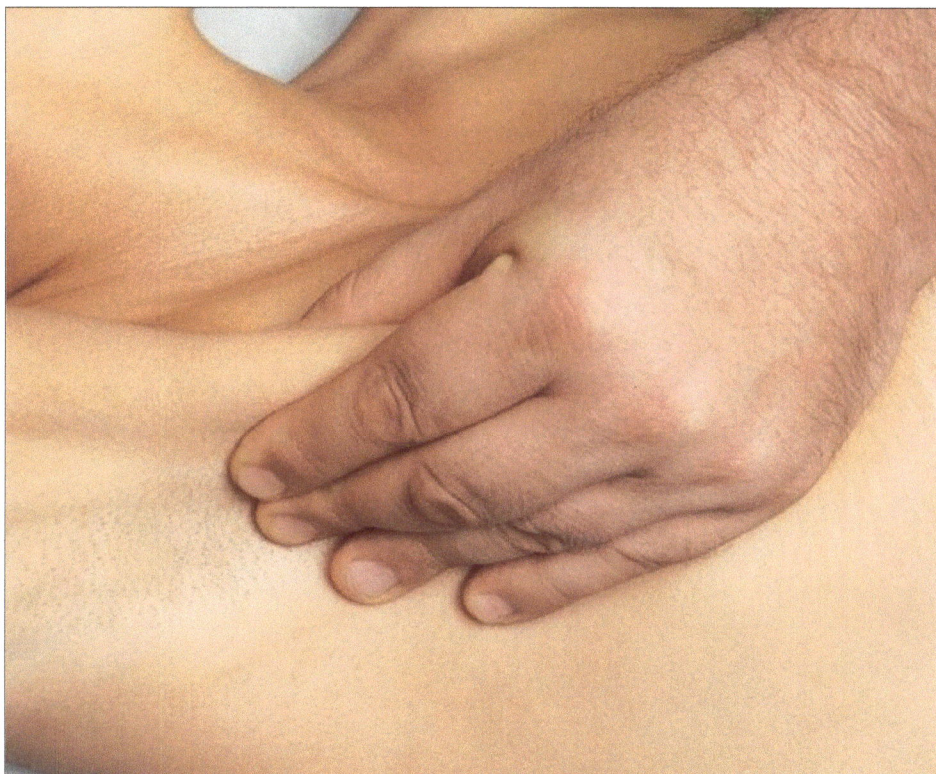

- ## Mammogram screening findings

  Mammographic changes as calcification it may indicate early development of breast cancer. Benign breast calcification can be excluded by biopsy.

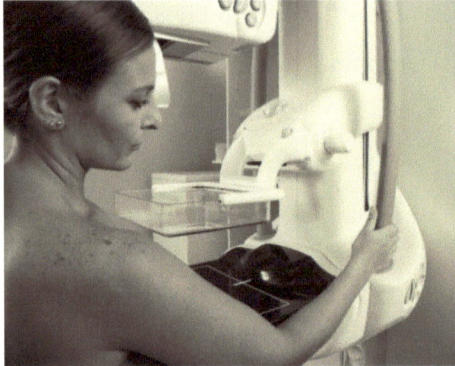

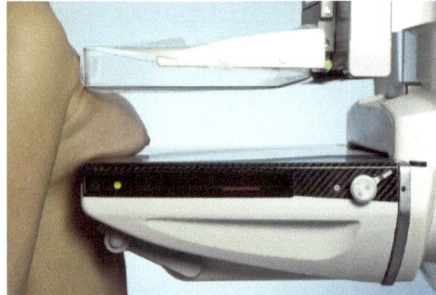

- ## Metastatic symptoms

  Breast cancer cells may spread before it appears as a lump or in skin changes and gives symptoms at metastatic sites as bone, liver, lung and possibly brain.

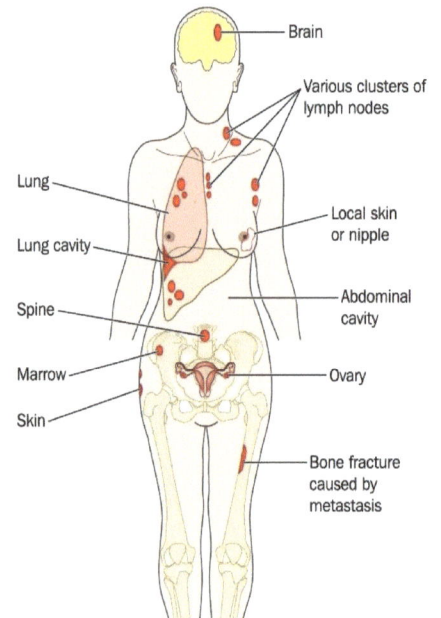

Breast cancer screening

Death from breast cancer has been reduced dramatically after early breast cancer detection with screening. Breast screening is normally started from early development of the breast at age 20.

A) Breast self-examination

Breast Self-Examination is the cheapest and easiest way of early detection of breast cancer. It is started from age 20. Breast self-examination should be done every month after 2-3 days of menstruation in premenopausal women, or at exact time of the month in post-menopausal women (refer on how to do self-breast examination later on page 16 of this booklet).

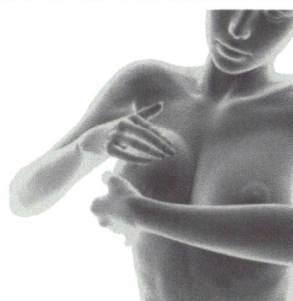

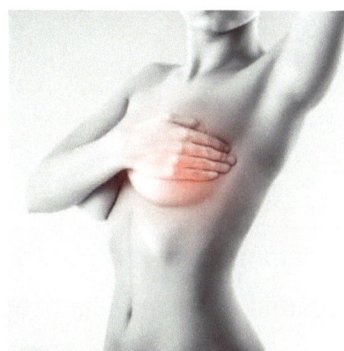

B) Breast examination by family doctor

Physician conducted breast exam is usually started at age 40, possibly even earlier if you are a high risk of breast cancer (refer to risk factor of breast cancer at page 21) or if you notice any breast changes during self-examination. If your doctor suspects any sign of cancer a further investigation will be requested as breast imaging and biopsy.

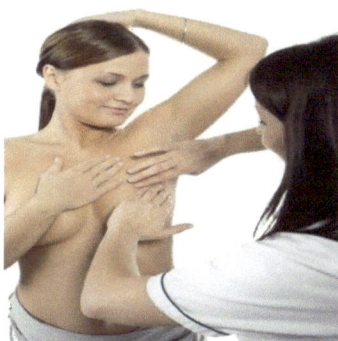

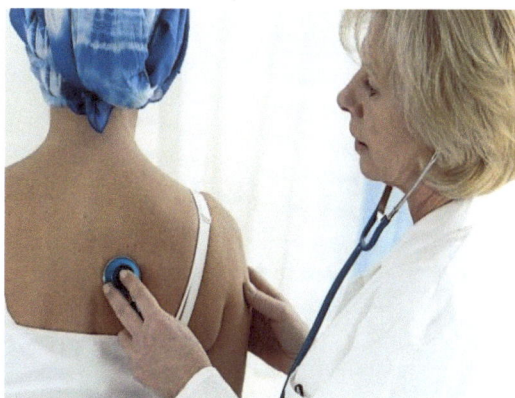

A patient's guide and explanations of Breast cancer treatment

Mammogram

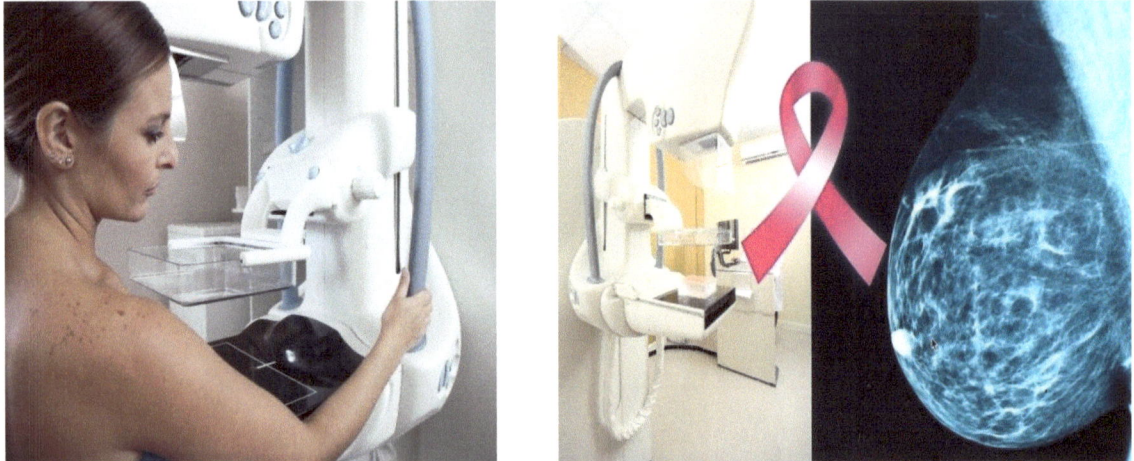

Mammogram is one of the most important methods for breast cancer screening. The mammogram is started at age 40 or 5 years earlier if a relative had developed breast or ovarian cancer. Mammogram is usually done on different views for better visualization with or without ultrasound of breast. You may be asked for breast Biopsy during screening if cancer needs to be excluded.

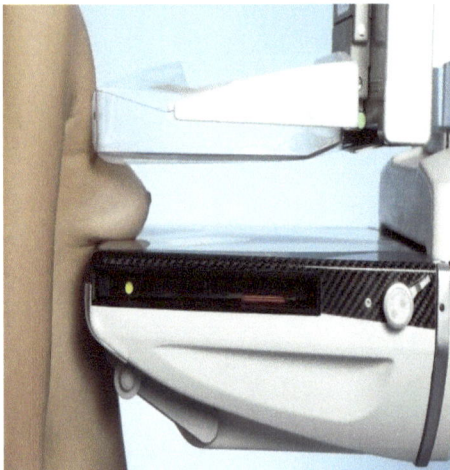

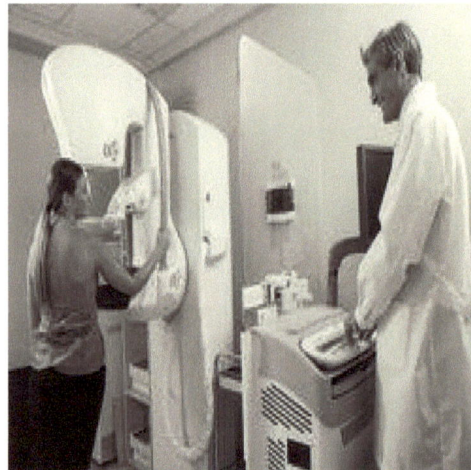

Magnetic resonance imaging (MRI)

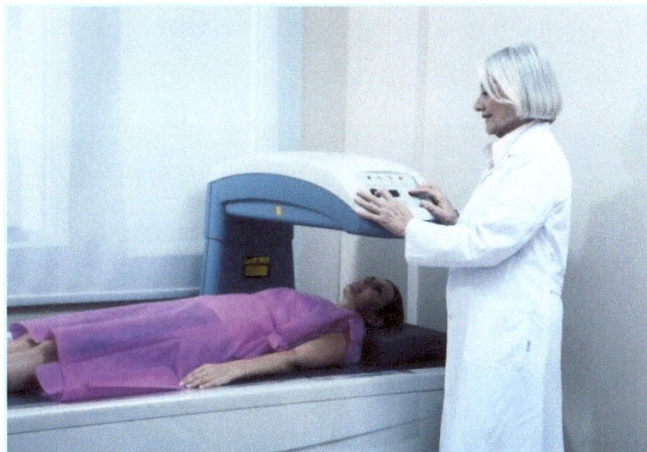

An MRI is rarely needed for breast cancer screening. The MRI may needed for patients when mammogram is un-safe to use, such as during pregnancy; patients with breast implant; when the mammogram is not clear due to previous reconstruction surgery, or negative with proven spreading of malignant cells to arm pit or to other parts of the body or prove to have lobular carcinoma.

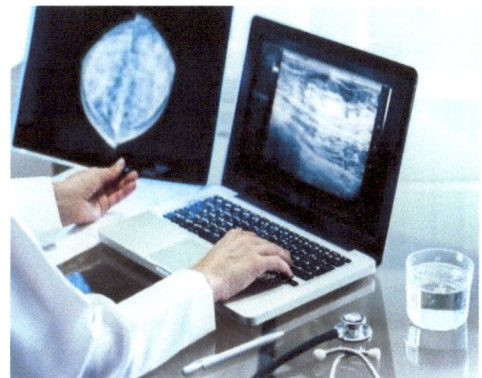

How to do breast self-examination

It is important to remember that breast self-examination needs to be started at early age when breast gland is developed, approximately by the age of 20.   If you notice any changes in breast than usual, go to your family doctor to examine you and if necessary, refer you for breast image or biopsy.

Keep yourself undressed from top until your waist, remove bra, shirt and any other clothing that covers your breasts.

1) Look at the mirror to both breasts

a) Keep your arms down and

- Compare if both breasts are symmetrical (similar to each other) in general size and shape.
- Look for any obvious lumps which can be visually noticed (without any touch)
- Skin changes (redness, dimpling, orange skin like, and ulcers)
- Nipple and areola changes (nipple retraction, nipple deviation, eczema like changes)

b) Raise your arms up and look for

- Any unnoticed lump in both breasts
- Look to the lower half of the breast and arm pit.

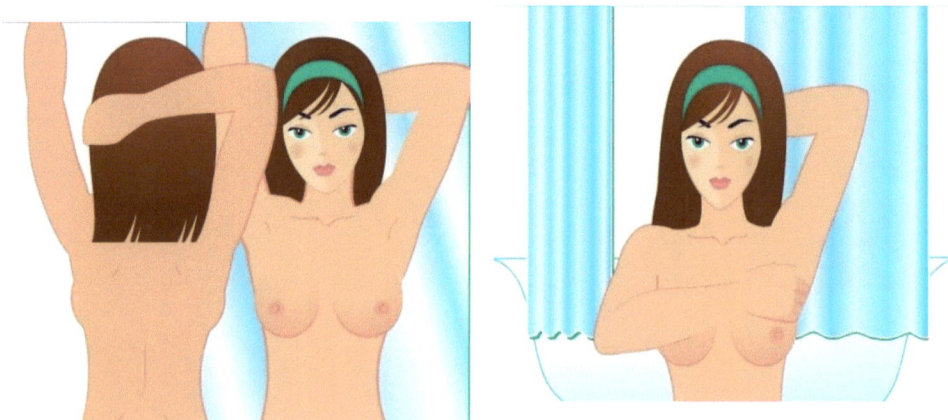

A patient's guide and explanations of Breast cancer treatment

2) Lay down on bed and keep small sheet folded under your shoulders (the reason for this is it raises the breasts and makes the examination easier).

Keep your right hand under your head and use the middle 3 finger tips of left hand to examine your right breast.

Examine the right breast by pressing the breast against chest wall in circular manner as clock wise until nipple areola complex, which needs to be examined by direct pressure to avoid missing lumps. Then examine breast tail under your arm pit.

Next, examine arm pit by keeping your arm down and relaxed, look for any lump both visually and by touch.

Repeat the same procedure with left breast by keeping left hand under your head and use right hand to examine the left breast and then left arm pit.

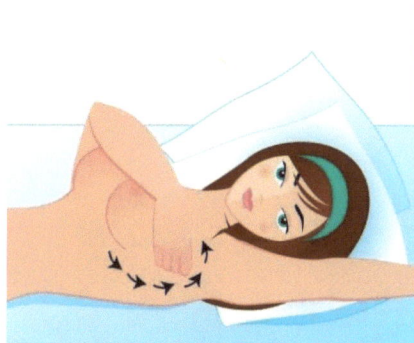

3) Check for nipple discharge on nipple

Massage your breast toward your nipple then press in your areola then nipple to encourage any underneath discharge. Often, many women have a normal discharge even without being pregnant of nursing. If this is normal for you, watch for any changes in discharge. If you have nipple discharge, it can be a sign of a potential breast problem. Look for discharge in your bra or clothing and report what you noticed to your physician as accurately as possible.

So, what is breast cancer?

Breast Cancer is defined as an abnormal cell that develops from breast tissue and grows at a fast rate and is capable of spreading to other parts of your body. Abnormal cells develop gradually by making small changes in the cells which make it different from its 'mother cell'.

That is why early detection of these changes can help to stop this abnormal cell to progress to cancer and spread.

Type of Breast cancer;

Glandular cancer:

Breast lobule :

1) Lobular carcinoma in situ is premalignant with high risk of developing of invasive breast cancer after 10 years. Usually discovered incidentally, and it is present in both breasts (mirror image), no surgery is needed, just you need close follow-up with MRI and biopsy.

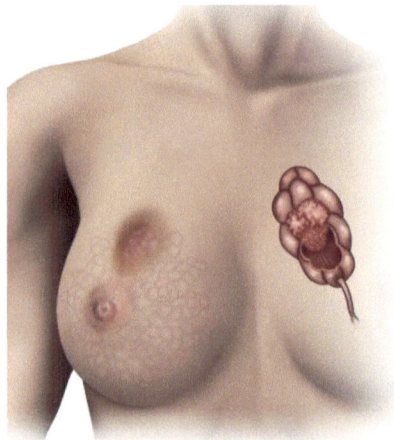

2) Invasive lobular carcinoma, cancer cell is originated from lobule and starts to go out of the lobule, medical, surgical treatment and radiation are needed.

Breast Duct;

1) Ductal carcinoma in situ, cancer cell is localized inside ducts and usually surgery with or without radiation is only treatment is needed

A patient's guide and explanations of Breast cancer treatment

2) Invasive ductal carcinoma is the most common cancer, when cancer starts to go out of the duct and it has high ability to spread to the lymph nodes and then to the whole body, this type needs medical therapy, surgery and may be radiation therapy.

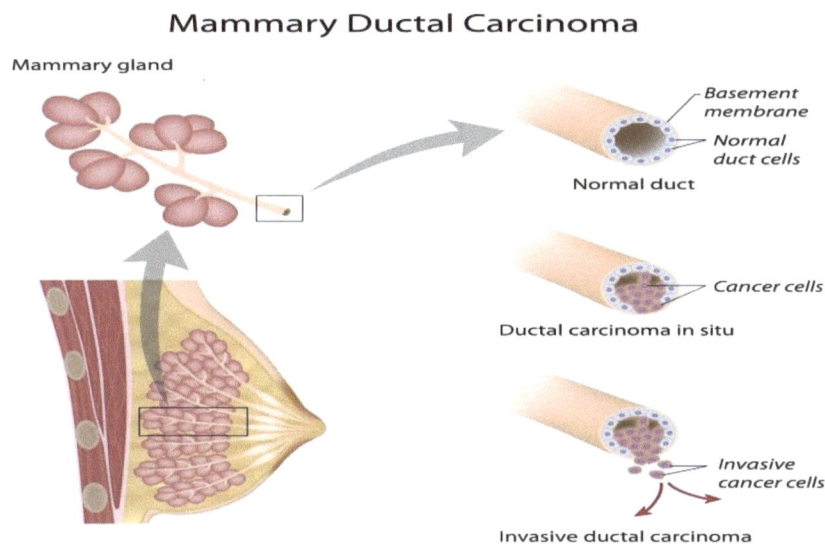

Mammary Ductal Carcinoma

Mammary gland

Basement membrane

Normal duct cells

Normal duct

Cancer cells

Ductal carcinoma in situ

Invasive cancer cells

Invasive ductal carcinoma

Learning points:

Carcinoma in situ means malignant cancer cells that have not migrated, spread or invaded other parts of the breast or other parts of the body.

Invasive cancer refers to a cancer growth that has the possibility to spread to other parts of the body.

A patient's guide and explanations of Breast cancer treatment

Others:

a) Blood vessels

Angiosarcoma is a rare malignancy, it is started from blood vessels inside the breast, sometimes originated by no apparent reason (primary cause) or possibly due to radiation therapy to the breast for previous lumpectomy (secondary cause). Usually it is noticed as a rapidly growing dark red or blue mass, rarely spreading to arm pit lymph nodes. A mastectomy is recommended because of it's high recurrence rate.

b) Lymph nodes

Lymphoma is a rare disease, it is part of whole body lymphatic channels disease. The most common treatment is radiation to the breast, surgery is rarely indicated or necessary.

c) Fibrous septum

Cystosarcoma Phylloides is rapidly growing tumor with high recurrence rate, need to be excluded from giant fibroadenoma by biopsy, rarely spreading out of the breast, recurrence rate is high, surgery is the only option.

Risk factors of breast cancer

- Early menarche (before 12 years old) and Late menopause (after 55 years old) make the breast exposed to female hormones (estrogen and progesterone) for longer time.
- No children
- Late age (after 30) at first birth
- Use of hormone replacement therapy long-term
- No Breast Feeding
- Personal history of lobular carcinoma in situ (LCIS)
- Personal history of atypical ductal hyperplasia
- Personal history of ovarian cancer
- Personal history of breast cancer
- Family history of breast cancer and/or ovarian cancer, particularly in a patient's first (sisters and mother) and second degree relatives (uncles and aunts).
- Personal or family history of mutation of the *BRCA1/BRCA2* genes.
- History of breast biopsy.
- Breast radiation

Note;

If there is any risk factor of breast cancer, it does not necessarily mean you will develop breast cancer but it is just you need to take more care than others.

Stages of breast cancer

The stage of breast cancer is indicate what level of breast cancer in your body

Stages of breast cancer
Stage 0
It is very early breast cancer and the cancer is still inside the duct or lobe with no tumor cells in the lymph nodes of the armpit.
Stage 1
Is an early breast cancer when cancer is small and starts to move out the duct or the lobule but is confined inside the breast with no skin changes and no tumor cells in the lymph nodes of the armpit.
Stage 2
It is a more advanced breast cancer than stage 1 with cancer cells starting to move to the lymph nodes in the armpit.
Stage 3
It is an advanced breast cancer with skin changes and lymph node involvement with cancer cells in the armpit.
Stage 4
It is a late breast cancer, when cancer cells start to spread to other parts of the body like bone, lung, liver, ovaries or brain

When to consult the doctor

- Breast or armpit lump
- Nipple discharge
- Nipple pulled inside or changed
- Eczema like appearance in areola and nipple
- Skin changes
- Newly developed asymmetry in the size of your breast.
- If you are at high risk of breast cancer
- Abnormal changes during mammogram screening.

You **must** immediately consult your doctor any time you find changes in your breast or in your armpit. <u>Don't ignore even the smallest lump in your breast</u> And remember to keep doing your breast self-examination.

Breast cancer evaluation:

Breast imaging

There are two types of imaging which are used for the breast evaluation: mammogram and ultrasound of the breast. These are used frequently, as it is difficult to determine the exact location and size of the lump and any other extra changes inside your breast that can't be felt. Sometimes the radiologist will ask for a biopsy to complete the lump evaluation.

Recommendations

Take shower on the day of your image and do not apply any lotion, cream, powder, deodorant, makeup, or perfume on your breasts and your armpit after your shower.

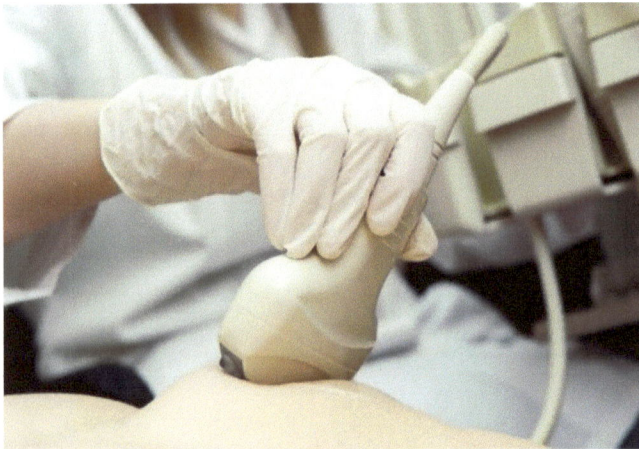

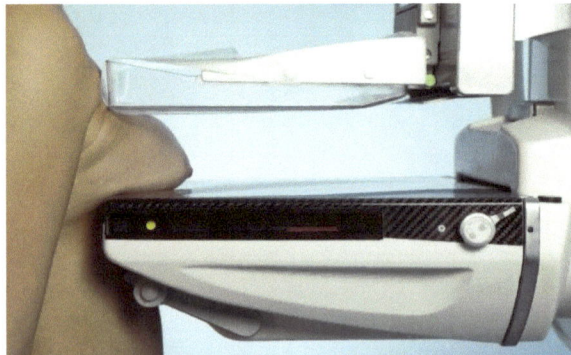

A patient's guide and explanations of Breast cancer treatment

Biopsy

When a lump is detected that may be cancerous, a biopsy is performed to confirm whether or not cancer is present and to provide information about the type of cancer that you may have. Your biopsy can be taken by a special needle and it is pain free as it will be taken under local anesthesia.

The radiologist will put a small metallic clip during the biopsy at the site of the lump to easily locate the lump later on. There is no harm from the clip and it can't be felt.

Recommendations

Inform your doctor if you are taking any blood thinner such as Aspirin, Warfarin or Heparin or Clexan.

After the biopsy, apply light pressure to the site of biopsy for few minutes in waiting area, if you feel pain you can take any pain killer.

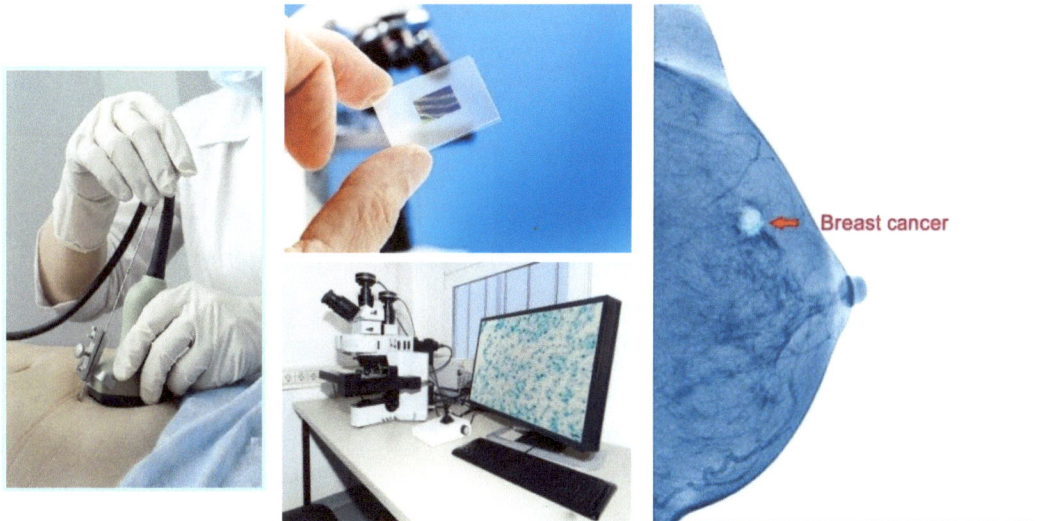

Breast cancer

Treatment of breast cancer

- ## Surgical treatment

All breast cancer needs surgery for breast and lymph nodes in armpit either before or after drugs. Sadly, a small number of patients can't go for surgery as they have a lot of comorbidities (serious chronic diseases) which may make general anesthesia a risk to their life.

Sometimes, the surgery is the only option for treatement; dicuss with your surgeon about your treatment options.

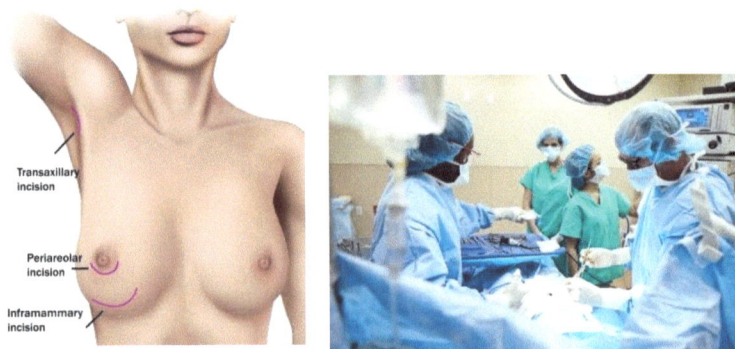

- ## Drug treatment

Drugs are used to destroy cancer cells in an effort to reduce the risk of your cancer coming back after surgery or making the tumor smaller and easier to remove by surgery. The type of drugs you will use depends on the type of cancer you have.   Your Medical Oncologist will discuss with you the treatment plan that you will need according to your pathology report.

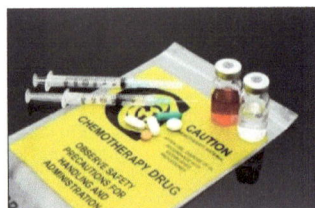

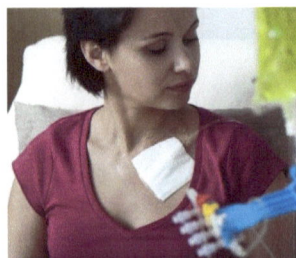

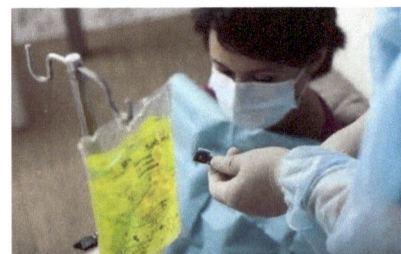

A patient's guide and explanations of Breast cancer treatment

▪ Radiation therapy

Radiation therapy is used after surgery to reduce risk of cancer returning. It is necessary in patients with partial breast surgery (lumpectomy) or If the breast cancer is advanced such as a large tumor or when the lymph nodes are involved.

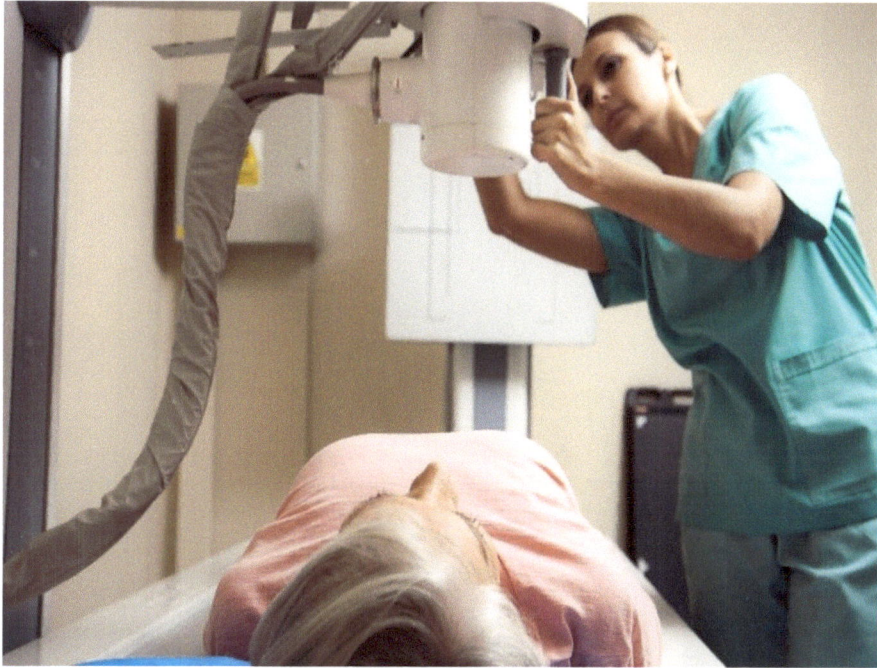

Surgical treatment of breast cancer

Surgical treatments of breast cancer

A) Surgery in Breast

I) Mastectomy

Removing all breast tissue.

Indications;

1. Large tumor (clinically or radiological)
2. Multiple tumors inside your breast
3. Unable to receive Radiation (pregnancy, history chest wall radiation, refuse radiation, disease in skin)
4. If lumpectomy will result in breast deformity
5. Some types of breast cancer such as inflammatory breast cancer and Paget's disease
   Note the risk of cancer reoccurrence is less than 5%

Types of mastectomy

a) Simple mastectomy (SM)

Is the removal of all breast tissue with overlying skin and nipple areola complex, scar is appeared as horizontal over chest wall, delay reconstructive surgery can be done after 1 years.

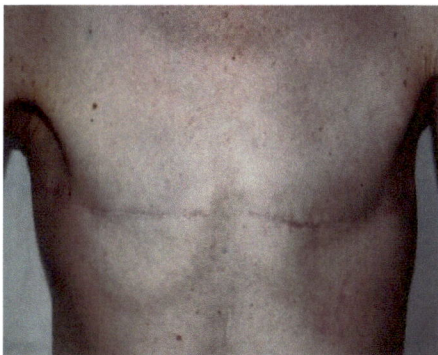

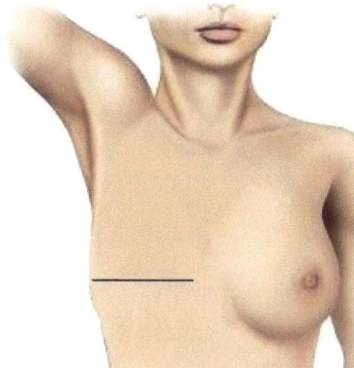

b) Skin sparing mastectomy (SSM)

Involves removing all breast tissue *without* overlying skin, the scar either horizontal or vertical and the pocket will be filled with implant or tissue expander (a fluid containing devise used to extend the overlying skin).

A patient's guide and explanations of Breast cancer treatment

- **Nipple sparing mastectomy** is removing all breast tissue *without* removing the overlying skin and the nipple areola complex

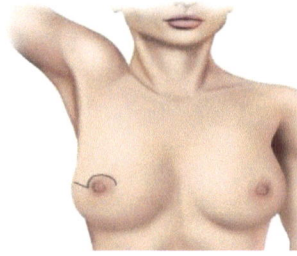

- **Non-nipple sparing mastectomy** is removing all breast tissue with nipple areola complex *without* removing of the overlying skin.

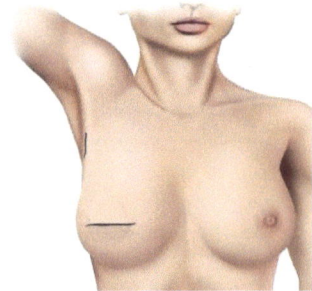

II) *Partial breast surgery:*

Definition;

Removal of the tumor with clear safety margins of normal breast tissue followed by radiation therapy.

Sometimes chemotherapy is given before surgery to reduce size of tumor and make it more suitable for lumpectomy.

Indications;

1. Small tumor found by examination and/or imaging.
2. Single tumor in the breast
3. Patient can take radiation treatment
4. The surgery won't cause any deformity in your breast

   Note   risk of breast cancer reoccurrence is 15-20%

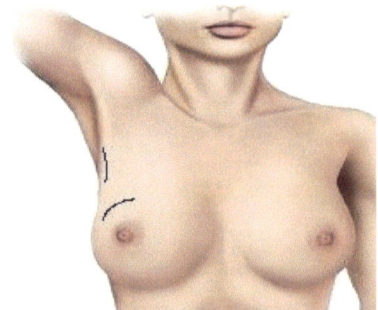

Types of partial breast surgery

a) **Lumpectomy or wide local excision**, remove the tumor with safety margin of normal breast tissue (no need for reconstructive surgery).

b) **Quadrectomy** removing all the breast quadrant,1/4 of breast size (requires immediate reconstructive surgery).

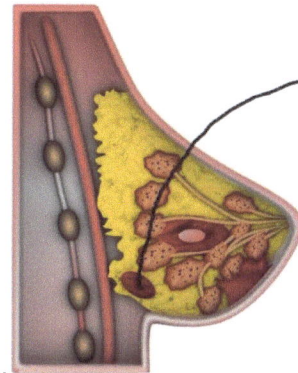

Some breast lumps are palpable for surgeon to remove during surgery but others are just seen on your mammogram and are often difficult too palpate by the surgeon.

There are two ways to locate non palpable lump ;
*First way, most common way is by using thin wire which is inserted at the center of the lump at the day of your surgery in radiology department before you go to surgery.
*Second way, is by using Radioactive seed, which is tiny as a grain of rice, and that will be inserted in the center of the lump in radiology department about one to two weeks before surgery. The seed containing lump will be removed by surgeon using special machine.

III) Reconstructive breast surgery

Reconstructive breast surgery is done to restore breast shape and size.

a) **Immediate reconstructive,** mean reconstruction can be done in the same surgery as with the breast cancer surgery to put either tissue expander (if radiation is planned) or silicone implant (if no radiation is planned) or by filling the space with breast tissue as in the Quadrectomy.

b) **Delayed reconstructive,** means reconstruction is done after the surgery of breast cancer, after completing the treatment, about 1 year or more using silicone implants or muscles to restore the breast shape.

A patient's guide and explanations of Breast cancer treatment

B) Armpit lymph node surgery

Armpit is easy to reach from the breast wound site so armpit lymph node surgery is usually accomplished at the same breast surgical wound site, but occasionally it may require an extra wound site in your armpit. This can be discussed with your surgeon about where your wound sites will be.

They are two types of armpit lymph node surgeries:

1. Armpit (Axillary) lymph node dissection

Remove all the lymph nodes from your armpit as it may contains tumor cells, and done as part of controlling the breast cancer.

2. Sentinel lymph node

Is the first lymph node that can receive the tumor cells. It can be detected during surgery to avoid unnecessarily Axillary lymph node dissection so future armpit surgery complications can be avoided (arm lymph edema and shoulder stiffness).

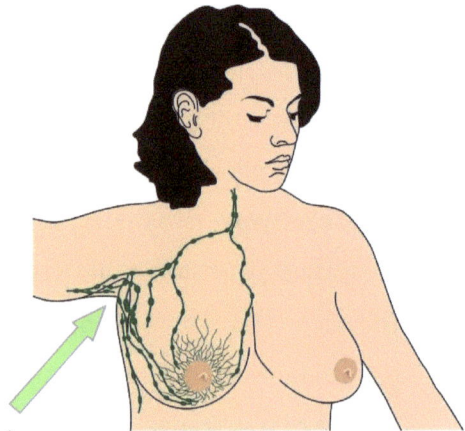

The sentinel lymph node can be detected by using gamma machine during surgery after injecting the areola with radioisotope material on the day of the surgery. The sentinel lymph node is removed during surgery and sent to pathology, it normally takes 15 - 20 minutes for the results to be known.

If no tumor cells are found in lymph node, no further surgery in your armpit is needed, if there is tumor cells found, an Axillary Dissection is needed while you are still under anesthesia.

C) Prophylactic breast surgery

Some people are very high risk to develop breast cancer in the future due to genetic breast cancer (BRCA1, BRCA2). Preventive surgery can be applied to these patients with immediate reconstructive surgery. Discuss with your surgeon for your concern and surgical options.

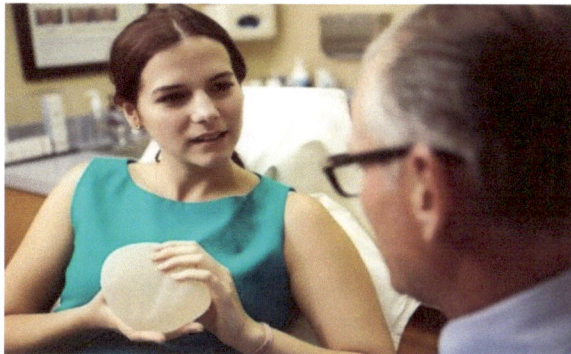

D) Prosthesis

For women who are not candidates for reconstruction on the same day as their breast surgery, there is a special breast prosthesis formed of silicon to be fitted inside the bra and give the matching appearance as the other breast. There is a different kind of prosthesis for one or both breasts with different texture and skin tones. Ask your doctor about these prostheses.

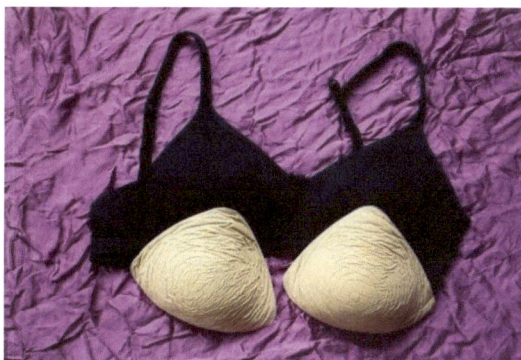

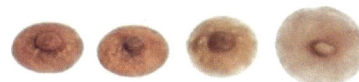

A patient's guide and explanations of Breast cancer treatment

Complications of surgery

- **Hematoma:** Accumulation of blood underneath the skin usually develops within the first 24 hours following surgery. Mild accumulation of blood doesn't require any surgical intervention but moderate and severe hematoma may need second surgery to evacuate this accumulation of blood.

- **Skin bruises:** change in skin color with bluish discoloration and this will resolve itself gradually.

- **Seroma:** the accumulation of serous fluid (clear, non-blood fluid) underneath the skin as part of body's reaction for the surgery, usually developing after 2 week of surgery and will be resolved within few months. Don't be concerned for this fluid as it **doesn't** mean that your cancer is returning.

- **Badly healed scar tissue (ugly scar):** is known as keloid or hypertrophic scar. It occurs in certain types of skin.

- **Wound infection:** showering before surgery, using antibiotics and control your blood sugar (if you are diabetic) can all reduce the risk of wound infection.

- **Shoulder stiffness:** or inability to move the shoulder joint due to Axillary dissection. This problem can be avoided by shoulder physiotherapy.

- **Winging of the scapula:** this very rare problem and occurs when nerve is injured during surgery or invaded possibly by the breast tumor.

- **Skin necrosis:** rarely happens but mainly occurs with very thin skin flaps and with smokers; the skin will first turn to blue then turns to black. Surgical removal of the dead skin is critical to do and then wound is closed later with skin graft.

- **Lymph edema:** accumulation of lymph fluid within your arm and that appears as a diffused swelling of the entire arm. It occurs as a complication of armpit lymph node surgery. Physiotherapy for your arm is needed to avoid such complications.

Drug treatment of breast cancer

Drug treatment of breast cancer

There are several drugs which are prescribed to cancer patients to be given as an outpatient. These drugs are helpful before surgery to improve the operability of the tumor and will help to reduce the size of the tumor and after surgery to kill any disseminated tumor cells in blood.

A) *Chemotherapy*

- This is an anti-cancer drug treatment used to kill cancer cells through whole your body, and it is given as during an outpatient visit through intravenous delivery.

- About 100 types of chemotherapy are used; your oncologist will use 2-3 types of drugs as combination in form of cycles for better effect.

- You will be seen first by your oncologist and review your pathology report to give you the right combination of chemotherapy, either it will be given before surgery or after surgery

- If you have decided on chemotherapy before surgery, usually it is given within 3 months in 2 - 4 week cycles, and some types may be used on a weekly basis. Several blood works and images may be required before chemotherapy is started.

- During the treatment, the response will be evaluated by your doctor so he will examine your breast to see if the tumor is shrinking and he/she may ask for further images, then you will be referred to the surgeon to do surgery after 3 weeks of the last dose of chemotherapy.

- If chemotherapy is given after surgery, it usually begins 2-3 weeks after recovery from surgery and before radiation treatment and it lasts for 3 months. During this chemotherapy treatment you will have regular blood work performed.

- The doctor may change the type of chemotherapy to another type if he notices no response or the disease gets worse.

- If your blood veins are hard to find, it can help to place a tube like called a "port-a-cath" (completely covered with skin and requires no care) or a "Hickman" catheter (hangs outside the chest) in a large vein. These devices are inserted by a surgeon and have an opening to the skin, allowing chemotherapy medications to be given, and it is safe to go home with until you finish your chemotherapy, then removed.

<u>**Helpful terms:**</u>

- Outpatient is when the patient goes to the hospital and leaves after the treatment, visit or procedure.
- Inpatient is when the patient goes to the hospital and stays over night or for a longer period of time.

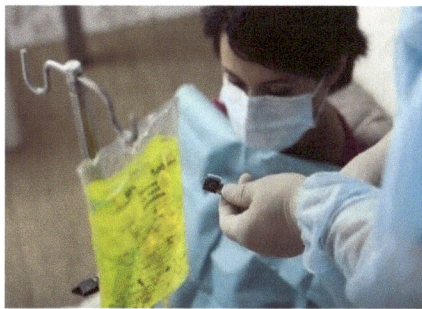

What do you expect after chemotherapy?

The list below is what you expect after you finish your chemotherapy. do not remain silent about what you are experiencing and tell your doctor or nurse about any complication you notice or feel.

- **Anemia** it will return to normal few months after chemotherapy.
- **Low white blood cells,** which make you more prone for infection; will improve after 3-4 weeks of last dose of chemotherapy.
- **Low platelets,** you will be more likely to bleed from gums, stool or with urine.
- **Hair loss;** is an obvious side effect of chemotherapy, hair follicles are one of sensitive cells to toxic effect of chemotherapy and hair will re-grow after few weeks of stopping your chemotherapy.
- **Nausea and vomiting** that will disappear after 3 weeks of last dose of chemotherapy.
- **Change in taste** that will return back to normal after few weeks (approximately 4 - 8 weeks).

A patient's guide and explanations of Breast cancer treatment

- **Fatigability** is because your muscle strength became weak. You will regain muscle strength gradually. Try to have daily walks with someone able to help if you need.

- **Numbness** that because of nerves are affected by chemotherapy but it will return after few months and it may takes a year because nerves re-grow very slowly

- **Nail changes** become more brittle, dark, and dry and are easily broken. Continue to cut your nail carefully without injuring your fingers and try to push cuticle (the tissue around the base of the nail) rather than cut it. It is important to avoid doing your nail in salon during this time due to the risk of infection. During chemotherapy, infections are difficult to heal – so avoid nail salons

- **Effect on the brain "Chemo-brain"** experiencing poor memory, inability to concentrate, unable to remember where you put your belongings. It is recommended that you always keep a notepad and pen nearby, write notes what you did and where you put your things. Have a family member or your spouse assist you during this time to help remind you and perhaps ask someone to be with you to help care for your family. Use a calendar to write your notes on. Do one task at a time. It may take several months after the chemotherapy for the chemo-brain effect to fade .

When do I have to go to emergency room?

- High body temperature greater than 38 degrees Celsius. Or if you experience fever and chills.

- New mouth sores or patches‹ a swollen tongue or bleeding gums.

- A dry, burning, scratchy, or "swollen" throat.

- A cough that is new or persistent and produces mucus.

- Changes in bladder function, including increased frequency or urgency to go, burning during urination, or blood in your urine.

- Changes in gastrointestinal function, including heartburn, nausea, vomiting, constipation, or diarrhea that lasts longer than two or three days or blood in stool.

B) Hormonal treatment:

Some of breast cancers are very sensitive to female hormones such as estrogen and progesterone and some forms of cancers are extremely sensitive to these hormones.

Some types of drugs (called 'hormonal therapy') are used to prevent the effect of estrogen to the tumor, causing the tumor to shrink and become smaller. It is given as an oral tablet before surgery if the patient can't tolerate chemotherapy. For post-menopausal women hormonal treatments continue for 6 months with frequent visits with the oncologist to do physicals and image examinations to evaluate the response to hormonal treatment. Hormonal therapy may be given after surgery for 5 years to 10 years to reduce risk of cancer reoccurring on same breast and on the other breast.

Side effect of hormonal treatment;

- Menopausal symptoms such as hot flashes, night sweats, heart palpitations, anxiety, sleep disturbance and fatigue may occur.
- Joint stiffness, pain and vaginal dryness may occur.
- Endometrial cancer
- Bone loss, which can result in bone fractures and osteoporosis. Your doctor may recommend that you have a bone mineral density scan, before starting your treatment. You may also need calcium and Vitamin D supplement.

C) Targeted therapy:

Currently there are two types of targeted therapy available in hospitals which are Herceptin (also known as Trastuzumab) and Tykerb (lapatinib). Both are highly successful in patients with positive HER2 receptors breast cancer. These are usually given intravenously with chemotherapy before or after surgery.

Follow-up with your oncologist

After you finish your medical treatment, your oncologist will follow you on regular bases for 5 years to10 years.

In every visit your oncologist will ask you if you have any new complaints. Make sure you tell him anything you have noticed! Tell the doctor all your concerns and questions, do not feel embarrassed and remain silent. He will request blood work and images for your next visit.

Follow-up with your primary physician near your home and update him / her about your conditions and follow for blood pressure, blood sugar, cholesterol, or infections that you may develop.

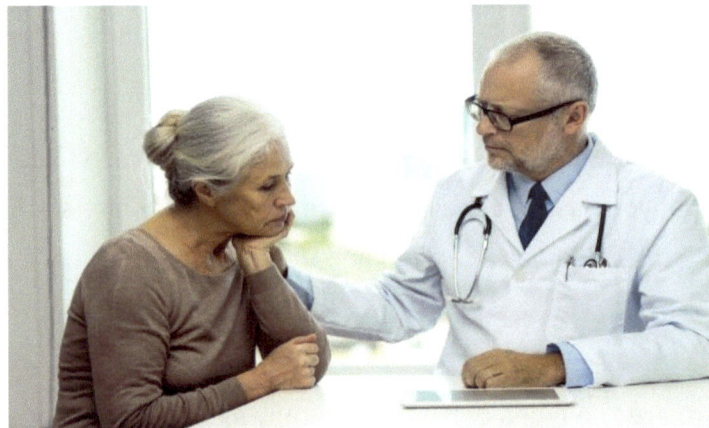

A patient's guide and explanations of Breast cancer treatment

Radiation therapy for breast cancer

A patient's guide and explanations of Breast cancer treatment

Radiation therapy for breast cancer

Radiotherapy is an external high energy radiation used to destroy cancer cells; to reduce the risk of breast cancer coming back in the breast, chest or lymph nodes. Despite the name, radiotherapy is not radioactive so it is safe to be with your children and your family after each day's treatment.

Do all breast cancer patients need radiation therapy?

No, some patients need radiation therapy as following;

1) After breast-conserving surgery

If you have breast-conserving surgery, you will be advised to have radiotherapy to the breast about 1 month after your operation, unless you're having chemotherapy, radiotherapy will be followed after chemotherapy.

2) After a mastectomy

Some women have radiotherapy after a mastectomy If:

- the cancer was large or aggressive
- there were cancer cells close to the edges of the removed breast tissue

3) To the lymph nodes

If the surgeon removed some lymph nodes from your armpit and they contained cancer

How the radiation therapy is given?

The treatment by radiation therapy is given in the hospital in radiation department on daily basis over a 6 week period; each treatment is taking about 15-20 minutes, throughout the week with a break over the weekend.

On your first visit to the radiotherapy department, you'll be asked to have a CT scan or lie under a machine called a simulator, which takes x-rays of the area to be treated. And usually you will have markings made on your skin to show the exact place where the radiographers (the individuals who give you your treatment) will direct the rays. Usually, permanent markings are made (tattoos). They're only done with your permission. It can feel a little uncomfortable while being made, but it ensures the treatment is given to the right area.

Your doctor will explain to you on your first visit about how the radiation will be administered and what the possible side effects exist. Make sure you ask any questions it may concern you and if you are pregnant you must notify your doctor before radiation is started.

How will I start my radiation sessions?

At the beginning of each session, the radiographer will position you carefully on the couch and make sure you are comfortable. During your treatment, you'll be alone in the room, but you can talk to the radiographer over an intercom, who will be watching you from the next room. Radiotherapy is not painful, but you will have to lie still for a few minutes during the treatment.

Current procedures are now applying Intraoperative radiation in which the radiation is given same time of your breast surgery for 30-50 minutes, however, this is only for older female patients with very early breast cancer.

What are the Side effects of radiotherapy?

You may develop side effects over the course of your treatment and that will disappear gradually over a few weeks up to a few months after treatment finishes. You will be given an appointment after each session in the clinic to observe side effects of the treatment. **Make sure** you let them to know about any side effects you have during or after treatment.

1) Skin irritation and erthema

Your skin in the treated area may get red, dry and itchy. Dark skin may get darker or have a blue or black tinge. If it becomes sore, your doctor can prescribe creams or dressings to help this. Skin reactions settle down 2–4 weeks after radiotherapy.

Here are some tips to help with skin irritation:

- Wear loose clothing not to irritate your skin, cotton fabrics are preferred .
- Have a shower but don't use any shampoo or soap, and avoid using any spray or deodorant if arm pit is involved.
- Pat the area gently and don't rub it with the towel
- Don't put anything on your skin in the treated area without consulting your doctor first.
- Avoid exposing the radiated area to the sun after treatment and use sun screen with SPF more than 50 .

2) Tiredness

This is a common side effect that may last up to a month or two after treatment. Try to get plenty of rest and pace yourself. Balance this with some physical activity, such as short walks, which will give you more energy.

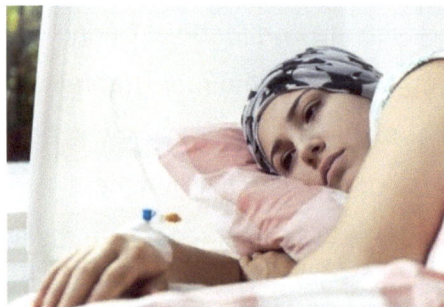

3) Aches and swelling

You may have a dull ache or shooting pains in the breast that last a few seconds or minutes and / or your breast may become swollen. These aches and swelling are to be expected and common.

4) Other side effects

Radiotherapy to the breast may cause side effects that occur months or longer after radiotherapy.

- Change in the look and feel of your breast and it become smaller and more firm and leather like feelings.
- Small blood vessels in the skin can be damaged causing red 'spidery' marks (telangiectasia) to show.
- Cancer in blood vessels of the breast (Angiosarcoma) but that is rare.
- It's rare for radiotherapy to cause any heart or lung problems or problems with the ribs in the treated area.

Your way for successful treatment

What do you expect on the first clinic visit?

1. Your first visit will be to **combined breast clinic** . First thing you do is go to the reception station and confirm you presence. Be sure to bring all reports and pathology slides if the biopsy was done outside. It is good to wear comfortable clothes to every visit with zip on top to be easy to approach your both breasts.

2. Your vital signs will be taken first in **nurse clinic**, and then you will be seen by **Breast Coordinator** who will take your personal information. They will need working telephone contact numbers (make sure they are active). It is good to give more than one correct contact number to make it easier to contact you.

3. A group of doctors including medical doctor (Oncologist), surgeon and radiation doctor (Radiologist) will see you and they will take complete history and do physical examination then arrange for you some investigations as blood work, imagines, and biopsy which can be done on same day or following day.

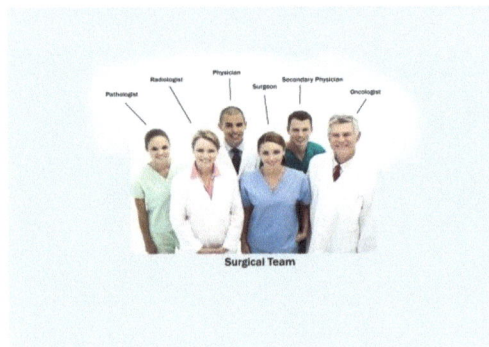

Surgical Team

4. The doctors will have meeting to discuss your case and develop your exact management plan.

5. You will be contacted by the Breast Coordinator who will tell you the new appointment either with the Oncologist, if chemotherapy will be started first or with the Surgeon, if surgery will be started first. You will visit the appropriate doctor and will give you the management plan designed for your case.

Meet your Surgeon:

- If you are suitable for surgical treatment or you finished the Neoadjuvant systemic therapy, surgical options will be discussed with you in the Breast Surgery Clinic in a very clear manner with all possible complications and alternative procedures explained and all your answers addressed. Upon gaining your consent for the intended procedure, you will be scheduled for surgery within one month <u>or</u> three weeks from the last dose of Neoadjuvant chemotherapy.

- **Make sure to write your notes with drawings on the back of this booklet.**

- Pre-surgical workups include blood work, electrocardiogram (ECG), appointment with Anesthesia and day of admission and surgery will be arranged.

Meet With Your Anesthesiologist

He or she will evaluate your general condition and if you are fit for surgery. The Anesthesiologist review all you medication and discuss with you the kind of anesthesia you will need

---

IMPORTANT!

It is very important that you read and understand the following!

Please tell us if you are:

- Taking a blood thinner. Aspirin, heparin, warfarin (Coumadin®), clopidogrel (Plavix®), and tinzaparin (Innohep®). There are others, <u>so be sure your doctor knows all the medications you're taking</u>.
- Taking prescription medications.
- Taking herbs, vitamins, minerals, natural or other home remedies.
- Having a cardiac problem.
- Having breathing problems.
- Experienced problems with anesthesia in the past.
- Having allergies, including latex.
- Smoking.
- Pregnant.

Preparing for your surgery

How to be ready for my surgery?

Preventing Pregnancy

Pregnancy can affect the path of your treatment and have a negative impact on your pregnancy, be sure you use birth control that does not have hormones, like a male condom, a diaphragm, or a Copper IUD. Or discuss with your gynecologist for your best birth control option.

Continue using birth control for about 1 year after treatment and then ask your oncologist if you plan to have children.

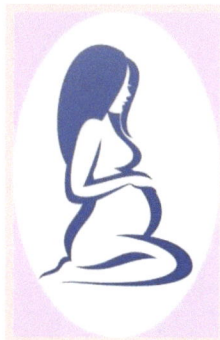

Stop smoking

Smoking affects your general health, do not think it doesn't – it does! In particularly smoking affects your breathing, it is mandatory to stop smoking for at least 10 days before your surgery!

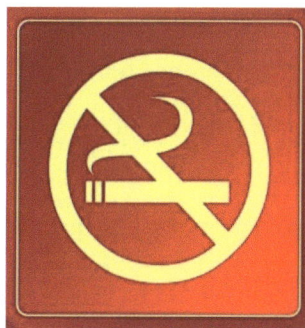

Have someone with you

It is preferred to bring someone (one person) with you during your admission for surgery and when you go home. <u>Children are not allowed to accompany you; please keep your children at home with a responsible adult.</u>

A patient's guide and explanations of Breast cancer treatment

Stop taking these medications

Here are some drugs you need to stop 10 days before your surgery, if you have problem in your heart or you develop thrombosis in your leg or brain, please consult your doctor.

- Any and all medications containing non-steroidal, anti-inflammatory drugs (NSAID) such as Aspirin.
- Blood thinners as Heparin, Warferin, Clexan.
- All medication containing vitamin E

Two days before surgery:

Take shower using an antiseptic soap or cleanser for your breast and armpit the day before and the morning of your surgery and that will help to reduce the risk of wound infection.

Leave all your valuables, such as credit cards, jewelry, and your checkbook at home

What to bring with you:

- Bring loose tops and comfortable pants or skirts or robe and cotton underwear and change for 2-3 days
- Comfortable shoes when you leave the hospital and while on your visit.
- Hand, facial cream and makeup as necessary.
- Personal Hygienic kit
  (Shampoo, conditioner, tooth brush, Tooth paste, hand soap, sanitary bag and pads)
- Hairbrush
- Cell charger with adapter.
- If your phone is pre-paid billing, ensure adequate credit is on your phone. If your phone is post-paid, ensure the bill is paid and will not expire during your stay.
- Book, magazines, IPod, notebook and pens.

One day before surgery

(If you have been planned to be admitted one day before)

- You will go to the Admission area and complete your admission process, then you will be guided you to your room.

- When you are admitted to your room, your assigned nurse will take brief information from you. Shortly after that, you will be examined by Breast Doctors and the procedure will be explained to sign the surgical consent, discuss all your concerns with the doctors. These are the same procedures explained to you by your Surgeon as described on page 47 (**Meet your Surgeon**).

- If reconstructive surgery was planned, you will be seen by the Plastic Surgeon and do drawing on your breast.

- The night before your surgery, shower using antiseptic solution or soap. Rub gently over your body from your neck to your waist and rinse. Do not let the solution or soap get into your eyes, ears, mouth, or genital area. Dry with a clean towel after your shower. Do not put on any lotion, cream, powder, deodorant, makeup, or perfume after your shower.

- Your doctor will use marking pen to do surgical site marking.

- Do not eat or drink anything after 12 midnight (the night of your surgery)

- If you are the first on the surgical list next morning and you planned for sentinel lymph node biopsy, you will be asked to sign consent and then you will go to radiology department before 4:30 PM the day before surgery to do injection then you come back to your room again. But If you are not the first on the surgical list then you will go to radiology department at 7:30 AM on the morning of surgery to do injection then you come back to your room or go directly to the operating room.

Day of surgery

(If you have been planned for admission on same day surgery (DSU))

- If you have been planned for same day surgery, make sure someone comes with you and will be there to take you home.

- You should be fasting at home at 12 midnight, <u>no drinking</u> or <u>eating</u> is permitted.

- Go to the Admission Office 6:00 AM and admission process will be done for you.

- Next, you will go to Day Surgery Unit (DSU). Present your admission papers to the reception at DSU and your nurse will guide you to your bed.

- You will be given: a gown, shoes, a cover and a cap and Your will be called for your surgery at 7:30 AM

Morning of surgery

- Do not put on any lotion, cream, powder, deodorant, makeup, or perfume after last shower.

- Do not wear any metal objects. Remove all jewelry, including <u>all</u> body piercings. The equipment used during your surgery can cause burns if it touches metal.

- Before you are taken into the operating room, you will need to remove your eyeglasses, hearing aid(s), dentures, prosthetic device(s) and any accessories.

- If your tumor is not palpable and lumpectomy was planned, you will be sent to radiology department when small wire will be inserted by image, to guide the doctor about the location of your tumor.

- Take your regular medications for hypertension, cardiac or thyroid with sips of water provided by your assigned nurse.

- Antibiotics will be given intravenously at the time of calling for surgery.

- Evacuate your bladder before you go to operation room.

- Wear your gown, head and shoe cover and stocking.

- Remove your contact lenses, hair clips, accessories, nail polish and underwear, if you have menstruation use disposable or cotton underwear.

Wire localization for non-palpable tumor

Before the procedure:

- On the morning of your surgery take shower

- **Do not put on any lotion, cream, powder, deodorant, makeup or perfume**.

- You will wear the hospital gown, make sure it is loose on you

During the procedure:

- The procedure will be done in radiology department in mammogram room by the Radiology doctor.

- Your breast will be assessed with ultrasound and/or mammogram and find the good place to insert the needle.

- Local anesthesia is applied to make the insertion painless

- The needle is inserted inside the breast

- Another film image will be taken to confirm the needle's location

- The needle will be removed and the wire will stay in place and covered by dressing.

After the procedure;

- You will go to your room or directly to the operating room

- Try to avoid any unnecessary motions to your breast to avoid potential wire displacement.

- The wire will be removed by surgeon during surgery with targeted lump

A patient's guide and explanations of Breast cancer treatment

Radioactive seed localization for non-palpable tumor

The procedure is done 1-2 weeks before surgery

Before the procedure:

- On the morning of your procedure take shower
- **Do not put on any lotion, cream, powder, deodorant, makeup or perfume**.
- You will wear the hospital gown.

During the procedure:

- The procedure will be done in radiology department in mammogram room by the Radiology doctor.
- Your breast will be assessed by ultrasound or mammogram and will find the good place to insert the needle.
- Local anesthesia is applied to make the insertion painless
- The needle is inserted inside the breast with radioactive seed (tiny as a grain of rice).
- Another film image will be taken to confirm the needle's location
- The needle will be removed and seed will stay at place inside the tumor and then the needle site will be covered with a dressing.

After the procedure;

- You will go to your home.
- You can do your regular daily routine.
- The seed will be removed by surgeon during surgery with targeted lump.

A patient's guide and explanations of Breast cancer treatment

Sentinel lymph node biopsy

Before the procedure:

- On the morning of your surgery take shower with antiseptic soap
- **Do not put on any lotion, cream, powder, deodorant, makeup or perfume**.
- You will wear the hospital gown, make sure it is loose on you

During the procedure:

- The procedure will be done in radiology department in nuclear medicine by the Radiology doctor.
- Your breast and areola will be cleaned with antiseptic solution.
- 4 Small injections of material will be injected under the skin of your areola.
- They will take films to your armpit to confirm uptake by lymph node

After the procedure:

- You will go to your room or directly to the operating room
- If you notice any rash, itching, shortness of breath, notify the nurse, as may you have an allergy.

A patient's guide and explanations of Breast cancer treatment

During surgery

- When you go to the operation room, your personal assistant (family member or friend) should confirm having an active cell phone, in case anyone involved in the surgery needs him / her. They can stay in your room or go to the cafeteria, as long as the cell phone remains on and a signal present.
- You will be received in operating room reception by the OR nurse where she will confirm your name, Medical Record Number (MRN), site of surgery. <u>Make sure you inform the nurse if you are pregnant or have any allergies</u>.
- During this time, your surgeon may still be busy with another patient. All your questions and concerns should have been asked before this time but if any questions or concerns arise, they may be asked.
- You will receive drug to make you sleeping before taking you to the operating room .
- In operating room you will be transferred to the operating table where you will started to sleep.

After surgery

1. After surgery you will stay in a recovery room (special room outside the operating room) to recovery from anesthesia for approximately 1 hour, after that you will be returned to your room or discharged if it was a day surgery procedure.
2. You will feel nauseated and vomiting for the first 24 hours because of the anesthesia drugs, you will receive something to reduce nausea and vomiting.
3. You will have pain at the site of the surgery, a pain killer will be given to you by IV and oral, please notify your assigned nurse if the pain is not controlled well or if you have allergy from that medications.
4. Nausea, vomiting and low grade fever is normal in first 24 hours after surgery.
5. You will feel pain in your throat because of intubation, it will be resolved within 24-48 hours
6. You will be fasting after surgery for 8-10 hours, after you wake up you can have clear fluids as instructed by your assigned nurse.

7. It is beneficial for early mobilization out of bed, then out of your room to avoid thrombosis in your leg. Ensure your personal assistant is with you during your mobilization periods.
8. Use small inhalation machine (Spirometer), it will be given to you or asked for it by assigned nurse and will teach you how to use it, use it 10 times/hour, and that will help you breath normally and to prevent you to have lung problems.

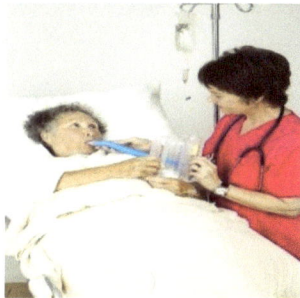

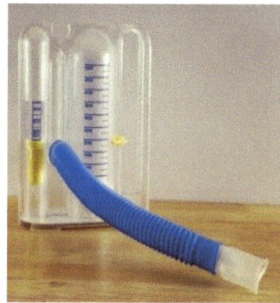

9. You will leave the hospital with at least one drain at outer side of your wound to drain the fluid collection and it can be removed when the fluid output is less than 30 ml/24 hours.
10. Avoid sleeping on the same side of surgery, and keep your arm on your pillow to avoid arm swelling if you had armpit surgery. If you want to get out from your bed turn to the unaffected side then rise your head and stay for few minutes before standing up.
11. Your wound will be closed with clips or stitches and covered with dressing which will be changed after 24-48 hours, or as soon as it become soaked after surgery.

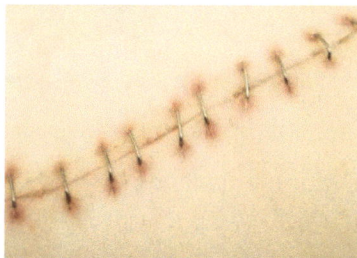

12. You will be visited by your doctor who will explain to you the exact procedure that was done and to see your dressing and drain.
13. There will be a steri-strips dressing over the wound, do not remove them.
14. You will receive antibiotics.
15. Discharge will be on the same day or within 24 to 48 hours of surgery unless your doctor asks you to stay longer.
16. Use your well fitted bra immediately after surgery if partial breast surgery (lumpectomy) was done and that is important to prevent hematoma formation.
17. You will be evaluated by physiotherapy nurse if surgery was performed in your arm pit.
18. You can have shower only after 24 hours of surgery.

A patient's guide and explanations of Breast cancer treatment

What do I expect after my surgery?

- You will be nauseated and may vomit after surgery, a special drug will be given to you to help.

- You will be drowsy for 6-8 hours because of anesthesia drug, take rest and sleep.

- If you have pain at the site of surgery, ask for more pain relievers.

- Throat is itchy and congested because of tube insertion, and that will resolved after 3 days.

- Numb or hyper sensitive skin at your surgery site and that will resolve after 3 months

- You feel your breast and nipple still there (phantom) that is normal and that will resolve after few months.

- Pain in your shoulder after armpit surgery; follow your physiotherapy instructions who will teach you simple moves to avoid stiff shoulder.

When I will be discharged from hospital?

- You should plan to be discharged from the hospital before noon the next day. You will receive a kit with the necessary dressing supplies.

- Most of the patients are discharged within 24-48 hours with drain, in reconstructive surgery you will discharge within 72 hours.

- Confirm you are taking your medications (pain reliever, antibiotics) and discharge summary.

- Make sure your supporter learn how to evacuate the drain, measure and document the drainage.

- <u>Don't use aspirin or Plavix or other blood thinner until you consult your doctor before discharge</u>

- All patients should receive an appointment before discharge in surgical clinic after 2 weeks, daily surgical wound nurse clinic for wound and drain care, after 3 weeks for clips removal and with physiotherapy clinic after1-2 week.

- If you want to wear an external prosthesis, it is better to use it only after 6 weeks of surgery.

- You can have your shower if discharge was decided and ask your assigned nurse to do dressing before you go home.
- Take your spirometry to use it at home for the next 3 days after surgery.
- Confirm to have sick leave from your day of admission until day of discharge with extra 1 month for the patient and 3 days for supporter / personal assistant.

After discharge:

During the first 48 hours after discharge you need to be in same hospital area , so if you develop any complications (like swelling of the wound, bleeding) you can be attended to promptly.

1. You will be seen on second day after discharge in the wound care clinic, you can take shower before coming to clinic for wound, drain care and reassurance.

2. On 5th day after surgery, you will be seen again in wound nurse clinic for drain output, review of the drain output documentation and check if the drain is ready to be removed. Usually, if the drain output is yellow and less than 30 ml in 24 hours, it is ready for removal.

3. After the drain is removed you need to start shoulder physiotherapy sessions to avoid shoulder stiffness.

4. It is normal to feel numb on your skin and on your arm pit; it will improved over several months.

5. After 3 weeks post-surgery, wound clips or stitches are removed

6. Avoid over using of affected side arm to avoid lymph edema and try to keep your arm at your heart level with pillow underneath your arm at side of surgery.

7. Avoid using the arm in same side of surgery for acupuncture and blood pressure cuff to reduce risk of lymph edema

8. If you notice that your hand is swollen after surgery try to keep 2 pillows and keep your arm above the level of your heart for at least 20-30 minutes or raise your hand above your head and close then open your fist slowly about 10 times. If the swelling is persistent or increases, consult your doctor on the first surgical visit.

A patient's guide and explanations of Breast cancer treatment

How to care about my wound

- The nurse will do change for your wounds before you go home. Keep the wound cover and ask for 3 extra dressings. The nurse will show you how to properly dress the wound.

- If your wound was soaked with a lot of blood while you are home, remove the dressing and apply new one without touching the wound, if you can't do that visit any nearby clinic and they can do that for you, if your dressing was persistently soaked, go to ER to exclude bleedings.

- Take shower while the wound is covered and apply plastic cover, and avoid rubbing with towel over the wound.

- You can take bath after 24 hours of surgery.

- If you have lumpectomy, fitted bra is preferred to use as soon as you arrive the room after surgery to avoid hematoma formation, and keep using the bra even at night time for at least 2 weeks.

- Apply gentle un-perfumed cream to moisturize the skin of chest wall.

- You may have 1 or 2 drains in use; a special form will be given to you from your assigned nurse and document the drain output, use this form in every visit with wound care nurse clinic until the drain in removed usually when output is less than 30 ml / 24 hours and yellowish color.

- You will learn how to evacuate the drain bottle by your nurse and you will have brochures about drains care (ask for it)

Consult your doctor if:

- You have a temperature 38.3°C or higher

- Your drainage (liquid coming out of your wound) increases, changes in color or consistency, or develops a bad odor.

- Your wound becomes red, warm or swollen.

- Your pain gets worse.

How to care of my surgery drain

After your surgery will have at least one plastic drain (tube with bulb) connected near your wound incision used to drain any fluid collection under your skin.

You will be discharged to home with this plastic drain, make sure to learn how to take care of it and how to measure the drainage with your assigned nurse.

1. Wash your hand with water and soap before and after handling your drain
2. Care about the drain site, the drain will be connected to your skin by tape, so avoid pulling or moving the drain away from you.
3. If you notice any thick clot in the line, gentile milking the line can help to remove the clot
4. Ask for family help to measure the drainage.
5. Measure the drainage twice daily ; open the measuring cup to be ready, open the bulb and don't touch inside it, pour the drainage inside the measuring container, then press on the bulb to create negative pressure then close the stopper ,discard the fluid in your toilette and rinse the cup with tap water for next use before your document the measurement(ml)
6. Repeat above steps when your bulb is full.
7. At the end of the day calculate the total of 24 hours for each drain separately.

After drain removal;

- Drain will be removed in the wound care clinic when the drainage becomes less than 30 ml; it is painless procedure, no need for anesthesia.
- Bandage will be applied to you after the removal.
- Extra alcohol swaps and bandages will be given for home cleaning.
- Keep the bandage for 24 hours.
- Take your shower
- Clean the drain site with alcohol swap then cover it with new bandage.
- Repeat this for 2 days then keep it open and dry because it is closed.

A patient's guide and explanations of Breast cancer treatment

Physiotherapy after breast surgery

Physiotherapy of your shoulders should be started on the 5th the day after your surgery and it is done if you underwent an armpit surgery.

Follow the examples in the figures below;

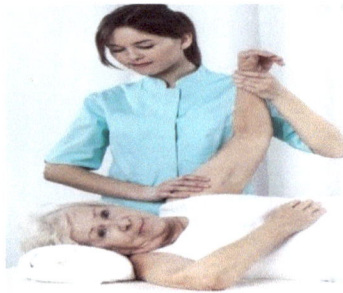

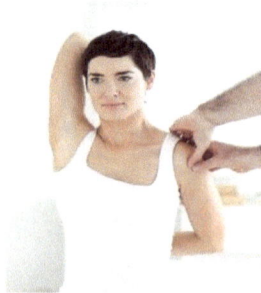

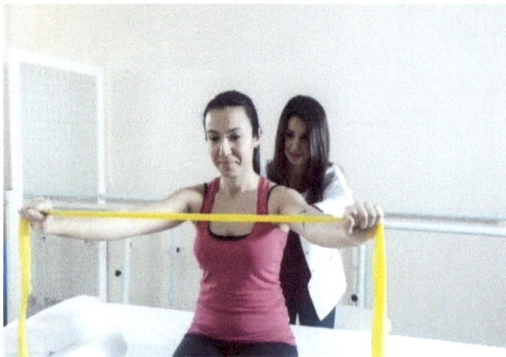

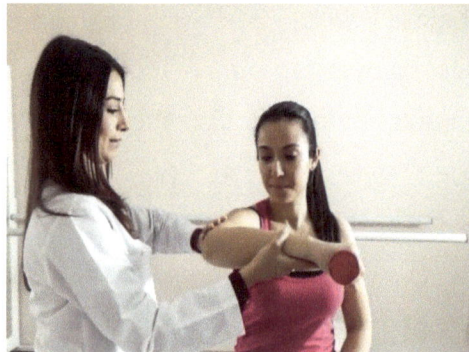

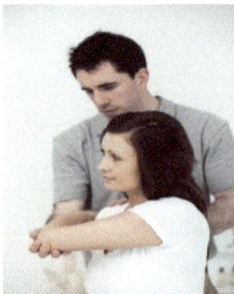

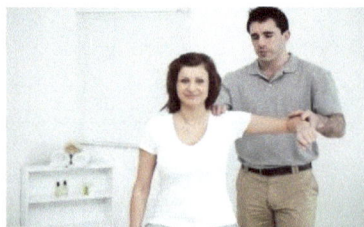

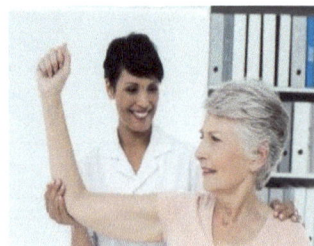

How to care about my arm after surgery;

It is important to take care of your arm after your armpit surgery because it is more prone for swelling (lymphadema).Physical therapists can treat lymph edema using a variety of techniques, including compression garments, exercise, and/or gentle massage.

- Avoid getting cut in the skin that can lead to infection of the affected arm.
  If you do get a cut, clean the area well and apply antibacterial ointment and a bandage. Watch the area for signs of infection until it heals.
- Use unperformed moisturizer daily to help protect the skin of your arm and hand.
- Clean your nails carefully. Do not cut the cuticles, just push it.
- Wear gloves when cleaning, or washing dishes and gardening.
- Use care when removing hair under your arm. Do not use a straight razor or hair removal (depilatory) cream, use the hair removal clipper.
- Avoid tight jewelry, clothing.
- Avoid over using of your affected arm as cleaning, pushing furniture, carry heavy groceries.
- Avoid blood drawing or the taking of blood pressures on the affected arm. If both arms are involved, use your feet as alternative place for blood drawing
- Use sunscreen with an SPF more than 50 to avoid sun burn in affected arm.
- Avoid the using hot bath; local heating and hot packs on the affected arm and shoulder.
- Cover your affected arm and hands when you are outdoor to avoid insect bite or use repellent spray if you are indoor

> **consult your doctor if:**
> - Visible swelling in the arm, hand, breast or chest.
> - Sensation of heaviness, achiness or tightness in the arm;
> - Easy fatigability of the arm or pain in the arm.

A patient's guide and explanations of Breast cancer treatment

Follow-up care

Follow-up after breast cancer treatment is necessary to detect and manage loco regional recurrence, distant metastases, new disease in other breast and treatment related complications, as well as dealing with reconstructive issues and psychological support. Follow-up visits are also designed to answer all of your concerns as well; so write all your questions and concern to be easy to remember when you visit your doctor.

1) You will be offered follow-up with surgical clinic after 2 weeks to check the wound and discuss your post-operative plan.

2) You will have more follow-up appointments with wound care nurse clinic for wound and drain care.

3) Visit wound care clinic if you develop any concern findings in your wound or drain.

4) You will have follow-up appointment with your plastic surgeon.

5) You will have an appointment with the drug doctor (oncologist) and the radiation doctor.

6) In all follow-up visits, keep wearing a comfortable dress or top can be opened in front with zip or buttons to make it easy to access the surgical site. This will relieve any unnecessary stretching to remove pull-over type shirts.

7) If you need medical report, ask your doctor for it in the next visit and in which language you need it , then you can receive it from medical report.

How to care about your breast after reconstructive surgery

After Your Surgery

- You will have gauze covering your wound this bandage will be held in place by your bra or clear tape.

- You may have two plastic drains in place when you leave the hospital. The drain is usually removed at your follow up appointment when your drainage is less than 30 ml, your nurse will teach you how to care for it.

- If you will be traveling by car, place a small pillow or towel between the seat belt and your reconstructed breast.

- The skin over your reconstructed breast is often thin and can easily be scraped which can lead to infection.

- If you have a loose gauze dressing, change in at least once a day.

- To create a natural fold under your breast, your surgeon may have closed your incision with stitches under the skin. These stitches dissolve and do not need to be removed. These stitches may cause you to feel a pinching or pulling sensation. This is normal and should not cause any pain.

Showering;

- Do not shower or wet your dressing for the first 24 hours after surgery. it can be covered with a clear waterproof cover, you may shower after 24-48 hours of your surgery.

- Avoid baths, hot tubs, and swimming pools for at least 6 weeks after your surgery.

- Avoid use deodorant, lotion, makeup, or cream anywhere nears your surgery site.

Clothing

- Wear a soft supportive bra for 6 to 8 weeks after your surgery.

- Wear your bra even while sleeping. You may remove your bra when you bath or shower.

- Do not wear a bra that has underwire.

- When you exercise wear a soft and supportive bra.

Exercise and activity

Avoid heavy activity that lead to overuse your chest muscles as swimming, tennis, riding horse and lifting for at least 8 weeks

Ask your surgeon if it is safe to resume your activates after 8 weeks.

A patient's guide and explanations of Breast cancer treatment

Tissue expander (expandable water containing implant)

After removing your breast, tissue expander will be applied under the muscle until you finish your treatment plan with radiation and keep stretching the skin to make new pocket to replace your removed breast (implant or muscle).

Special instruction for tissue expander;

- Your constructed breast looks smaller because it is not fully inflated.
- Ask your plastic surgeon to locate the port where he/she will use it for inflation.
- It needs frequent visit to inflate your tissue expander; you may feel discomfort for few days because of stretching your skin.
- Tissue expander has metallic, avoid using MRI.
- Ask for report from your surgeon about tissue expander as it will trigger the alarm in airport.

Consult your doctor if:

- A temperature of (38° C) or higher or chills.
- Redness, warmth or increased pain in the breast area
- Drainage or oozing from an incision
- Any type of skin infection on any part of your body need to take an antibiotic to avoid secondary infection on your implant.

PATIENT'S RIGHTS

EDUCATION AND INFORMATION BOOKLET

Many educational brochures' are available in clinics about breast cancer, take your time and collect some of them to read it at home. You will have an informational booklet with illustrations is available to help you to understand your disease and surgical plan, write your notes and questions on the back of the booklet.

MEDICAL REPORT

An updated medical report can be provided to you upon your request in surgical clinic inform the doctor where you want to present the report.

FLIGHT TICKETS AND ACCOMMODATIONS ARRANGMENT

If you are from outside where you will perform your surgery, arrange your flight tickets and accommodation after you discharge from hospital.

SICK LEAVE AND WORK EXCUSE;

Sick leave for the patient from the date of admission to the date of discharge with 1 month after discharge date.
Work excuse for your supporter from the date of admission to the date of discharge and 3 days extra after discharge to take care of you.

APPOINTMENTS AND MEDICATIONS.

Before you go home you will be provided with medications (pain killer and antibiotics), dressing supply and appointments with wound care clinic, physiotherapy and surgeon clinic, make sure to have all appointments before you leave the hospital.

A patient's guide and explanations of Breast cancer treatment

FREQUENTLY ASKED QUESTIONS (FAQ)

- **Is it normal to have nausea and vomiting after surgery?**

  Yes that is part of anesthesia effect in your body and that will resolve after 24 hours, you will be given medications to prevent it.

- **When I will be discharged after surgery?**

  You will be discharged same day or after 24 hours if there is reconstruction surgery was done

- **When I can take shower?**

  You can take your shower before you go home and before each visit to wound care nurse clinic, allow water to flow over the dressing without rubbing it.

- **Can I make religious pilgrimage?**

  Yes you can go for religious pilgrimage as soon as you feel you are able to do so.

- **Is it safe to do prayer immediately after surgery?**

  Yes you can pray as soon as you are awake from surgery.

- **Is it safe to travel as soon as I discharge from the hospital?**

  It is preferred to stay in hospital area for 48 hours.

- **Which is preferred to travel car or plane?**

  There is no difference; you can travel by the method you find it good for you.

- **Is there any place I can get breast prostheses?**

  Yes you can ask your nurse in clinic and she will guide you for it, or contact us at

  Email ; info@eid-otto.com

- **When I can wear my prostheses after surgery?**

  It is preferable to wear it after 6 weeks.

- **When I can know my histopathology report and if I need further treatment?**

  Your histopathology result and further treatment plan will be discussed in your first post operative visit in surgical clinic after 2 week from discharge.

- **If I have complication in the wound and my next appointment after 1 week where do I have to go?**

  You will have an appointment in wound care nurse clinic on next day morning after surgery, if you notice any change in the wound, visit your nurse in clinic if you have appointment or go to ER if you don't have appointment.

- **When the drain will be removed?**

  The drain can only be removed when the drain output less than 30 ml and clear and that is usually after 5 days of surgery.

- **Do all patients with breast cancer will receive chemotherapy?**

  No, some patient need chemotherapy and some don't need.

- **If I have Axillary lymph node metastases do I have to remove the rest of Axillary lymph nodes?**

  Yes you need to do an Axillary lymph node dissection but in some cases axillary surgery it may not needed, discuss this with your surgeon and medical oncologist.

- **Is it necessarily to have radiation therapy to my breast after surgery, and What is the complication of radiation therapy?**

  Not all patients need radiation therapy, indication and complication of radiation therapy see page 43.

- **What is the radioactive seed?**

  Radioactive seed is tiny as a grain of rice with very minimal radiation used to help the surgeon to locate non-palpable breast lump with special machine used during surgery, it is only used if you are for lumpectomy and the lump is difficult to fell by hand.

My treatment plan

My Name: _____MRN_____

Name of Surgeon: _____

Name of Oncologist: _____

Name of Radiation Oncologist: _____

Name of physiotherapist; _____

Your breast drawing here

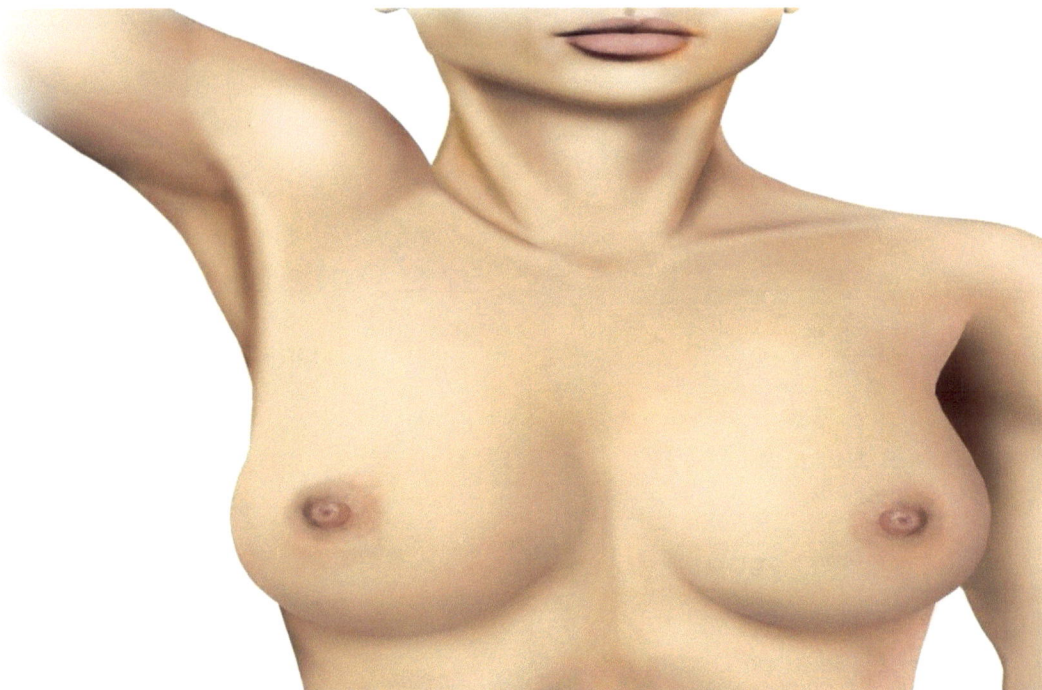

My Breast Surgery Notes

Tumor type_____ Tumor size_____ Tumor location _____

Hormonal receptors_____   HER2 receptors_____

Cancer stage _____   Date of surgery: MM / DD / YYYY

Treatment plan   ☐   Drugs   ☐   Surgery   ☐   Radiation

Type of surgery in breast: ☐   lumpectomy   ☐   mastectomy

Reconstruction   ☐ immediate   ☐   delayed   ☐   no reconstruction

Type of surgery in armpit ☐ sentinel lymph node ☐   LN dissection

Number of lymph node positive: _____   margins:-_____

Drugs therapy ☐ Chemotherapy ☐ Hormonal   ☐   Targeted therapy

A patient's guide and explanations of Breast cancer treatment

MY NOTES - QUESTIONS - CONCERNS

A patient's guide and explanations of Breast cancer treatment

Record of Drainage Output

Please bring with you this form in each wound care clinic

Date	morning		Evening		Total		Note
	Drain1	Drain2	Drain1	Drain2	Drain1	Drain2	

A patient's guide and explanations of Breast cancer treatment

Record of Drainage Output (continue)

Please bring with you this form in each wound care clinic

Date	morning		Evening		Total		Note
	Drain1	Drain2	Drain1	Drain2	Drain1	Drain2	

A patient's guide and explanations of Breast cancer treatment

Common Medications need to stop before surgery or breast biopsy.

The following are the medications that contain aspirin and other non steroidal anti-inflammatory drugs (NSAIDs). It's important to stop these medications before many surgery or biopsy because some medications can increase your risk of bleeding.
 Tell your doctor or nurse if taking these medications before your surgery or biopsy.

If you're having surgery:
Stop taking medications that contain aspirin or vitamin E 10 days before your surgery or as directed by your doctor. If you take aspirin because you've had a problem with your heart or you've had a stroke, be sure to talk with your doctor before you stop taking it. Stop taking NSAIDs 48 hours before your surgery.

Following are blood thinner need to get instruction by your doctor.

Coumadin   Heparin   Lovenox®   Persantine®   Plavix®   Pletal®

The following common medications contain aspirin need to stop it 10 days before surgery;

Alka Seltzer®
Anacin®
Arthritis Pain Formula
Arthritis Foundation
  Pain Reliever®
ASA Enseals®
ASA Suppositories®
Ascriptin® and
Ascriptin A/D®
Aspergum®
Asprimox®
Axotal®
Azdone®
Bayer® (most
formulations)
BC® Powder and
  Cold Formulations
Bufferin®
  (most formulations)
Buffets II®
Buffex®

Cama® Arthritis
  Pain Reliever
COPE®
Dasin®
Easprin®
Ecotrin (most
formulations)
Empirin® Aspirin
  (most formulations)
Epromate®
Equagesic Tablets
Equazine®
Excedrin® Extra-
  Strength Analgesic
  Tablets and Caplets
Excedrin® Migraine
Fiorgen ®
Fiorinal®
  (most formulations)
Fiortal®
Gelpirin®

Genprin®
Gensan®
Heartline®
Headrin®
Isollyl®
Lanorinal®
Lortab® ASA Tablets
Magnaprin®
Marnal®
Micrainin®
Momentum®
Norgesic Forte®
  (most formulations)
Norwich® Aspirin
PAC® Analgesic Tablets
Orphengesic®
Painaid®
Panasal®
Percodan® Tablets
Persistin®
Robaxisal® Tablets

Roxiprin®
Saleto®
Salocol®
Sodol®
Soma® Compound
Tablets
Soma® Compound
  with Codeine Tablets
St. Joseph® Adult
  Chewable Aspirin
Supac®
Synalgos® DC Capsules
Tenol-Plus®
Trigesic®
Talwin® Compound
Vanquish® Analgesic
  Caplets
Wesprin® Buffered
Zee-Seltzer®
ZORprin®

A patient's guide and explanations of Breast cancer treatment

The following common medications are NSAIDs that do not contain aspirin need to stop it 2 days before surgery:

Advil®	Children's Motrin®	Indomethacin	Mobic®	Piroxicam
Advil Migraine®	Clinoril®	Indocin®	Motrin®	Ponstel®
Aleve®	Daypro®	Ketoprofen	Nabumetone	Relafen®
Anaprox DS®	Diclofenac	Ketorolac	Nalfon®	Saleto 200®
Ansaid®	Etodolac®	Lodine®	Naproxen	Sulindac
Arthrotec®	Feldene®	Meclofenamate	Naprosyn®	Toradol®
Bayer® Select	Fenoprofen	Mefenamic Acid	Nuprin®	Voltaren®
Pain Relief	Flurbiprofen	Meloxicam	Orudis®	
Formula Caplets	Genpril®	Menadol®	Oxaprozin	
Celebrex®	Ibuprofen	Midol®	PediaCare Fever®	

Most multivitamins contain vitamin E, so if you take a multivitamin be sure to check the label. The following products contain vitamin E(less than 400 IU Daily is ok):

Amino-Opt-E	Aquavit	E-400 IU	E complex-600
Aquasol E	D'alpha E	E-1000 IU Softgels	Vita-Plus E

Supplements and Herbals to avoid 10 days before surgery.

Birch Bark	Turmeric	Chinese Black Tree Fungus	Cayenne	St. John's Wort
Cumin	Danshen	Ephedra/ Ephedrine	Primrose Oil	Feverfew
Garlic	Ginger	Ginko Biloba	Onion Extract	Goldenseal
Grape seed Extract	Kava	Ma Huang	Milk thistle	Omega 3 Fatty Acids

A patient's guide and explanations of Breast cancer treatment

Component	Time	Location	Note
Before surgery	First clinic visit	Breast clinic	• History and Physical exam • Images • Biopsy
	5th day	Doctors meeting	• Call you for appropriate clinic next week
	10th- -12th day	Surgical breast clinic	• If Surgery was planned surgical options will be discussed with you
		counselor clinic	• Questions and concerns
		Anesthesia clinic	• Assess your general condition • Bring all your medications
	Admission	Surgical ward	• stop some medication 10 days before surgery • take shower before admission • seen by surgeon • fasting at 12 Midnight
Surgery	Day 0 (day of surgery)	Surgical ward	• shower • seen by surgeons • sentinel injection • wire or radioactive seed localization • remove accessories ,jewelries ,piercings • Wear gown, cap. overshoes
		operating room	• inform the nurse if you have allergy
		Surgical ward	• fasting for 8 hours • sips of water under your nurse supervision • seen by surgeon • ambulation • spirometer • wound and drain care • pain control
After surgery	Day 1 (Discharge)	Surgical ward	• Drain care education • Physiotherapy • Ambulation • spirometer • Appointments and Medications • Social worker for accommodation and flight tickets
	Day 3	Wound care clinic	• take shower at home • Wound dressing • drain care • reassurance
	Day 5		• Drain removal (if less than 30ml) • Wound dressing
	Day 8		• Drain removal if not removed before • Wound dressing
		physiotherapy	• physiotherapy
follow-up	Day 15	Surgeon clinic	• check wound • discus your pathology result • Follow-up after 6 months.
	Day 22	Wound care nurse clinic	• Clips removal • wound care
	Day 30		• Confirm the Wound is healed. • Drain and clips are removed. • patient discharged

.SUMMARY OF YOUR PATHWAY IN BREAST SURGERY UNIT

A patient's guide and explanations of Breast cancer treatment

A patient's guide and explanations of Breast cancer treatment

www.ingramcontent.com/pod-product-compliance
Lightning Source LLC
Chambersburg PA
CBHW042015080426

42735CB00002B/59

9 780990 932208